Beyond superb! Clearly written Jones' beautiful story will surely struggling with chronic fatigue This book is one on its own. I can it highly enough for anyone whose life is being challenged by CFS. This book provides an easy-to-read story which educates not only about *what* to do, but also explains *why* to do it and shows *how* to do it! Her own story at the beginning brought me to tears... there is no better person to help others than someone who has gone through the experience themselves and found the light at the end of the tunnel. Charlotte Jones is that person... an absolute inspiration!
  – Lesley Una Pierce, director of The Nutritional Healing Foundation

A spectacular debut, perfect for those with CFS who want to regain their power.
  – Emily McGuire, living with chronic fatigue syndrome

This will be such an important book for health professionals who work with patients experiencing chronic pain or low energy. Empowering patients to understand how the body works in terms of positive and negative influences on their energy will be a powerful treatment tool to help give patients greater control over their health.
  – Angela Jackson, chartered physiotherapist

This is the first time I have read something about CFS that actually understands how I feel and more importantly how to change it, not written by someone who studied it but by someone who actually climbed out of the dark tunnel. This magical story made me smile but more importantly it's teaching me how to believe in myself, stop the negative cycle and finally climb out of my dark hole and change my life. I now truly believe that I am brave and strong.
  – Kim Sibley, living with chronic fatigue syndrome

From Fatigue to Freedom

An Inspiring Journey to Better Energy and Brighter Days

CHARLOTTE JONES

Illustrations by
Lynn Redwood
Instagram: @lynnredwoodart

From Fatigue to Freedom
ISBN 978-1-915483-12-6
eISBN 978-1-915483-13-3

Published in 2023 by Right Book Press
Printed in the UK

© Charlotte Jones 2023

The right of Charlotte Jones to be identified as the author of this work has been asserted in accordance with the Copyright, Designs and Patents Act 1988.

A CIP record of this book is available from the British Library.

All rights reserved. No part of this book may be reproduced, stored in a retrieval system, or transmitted in any form or by any means, electronic, mechanical, photocopying, recording or otherwise, without the prior written permission of the copyright holder..

This book is dedicated to my late mum Joanna and my husband Anthony, two people in my life who have always believed in me and to whom I am eternally grateful; to my two children, Georgie and Nick, who supported me with their care when I was ill and their enthusiasm while I was on my writing journey; and to my dad Jim, who has given me so much of his time to help me through the writing of this book; he has been pleasantly surprised and delighted that I have produced one!

Disclaimer

The information presented in this book is the author's opinion and does not constitute any health or medical advice. The content of this book is for informational purposes only and is not intended to diagnose, treat, cure or prevent any condition or disease. Please seek advice from your healthcare provider for your personal health concerns.

CONTENTS

Foreword by Professor Vinod Patel	ix
Angela's journey	xii
Introduction	1
1 **Hugo Hope and the magic marbles of energy**	11
Fight or flight and rest and repair	
2 **Barbara Bellows, Billie Bubble and Henry Happy**	23
Breathwork, a protective bubble and the importance of smiling	
3 **Clara Calm and Toby Time**	33
Pace yourself and define your day with moments of serenity	
4 **Felicity Food**	43
Think of food as your medicine	
5 **Nathan Night**	55
A good night's sleep helps the body to heal	
6 **Hana Habit and Milo Movement**	63
Healthy habits and movement to connect the mind and body	
7 **Harpreet Health**	75
A healthy gut rules the day	
8 **Herbie Holistic**	89
Understanding, nurturing and working with your body	
9 **The Butterfly Mountain**	99
10 **Making sense of it all**	109
Time to look at you	
The resources section	125
Explaining the why and how	
Glossary of terms	151
References and reading	161
Acknowledgements	167
About the author	170

FOREWORD

I feel honoured to have been given the opportunity to write a foreword for this interesting fable of how to manage and overcome chronic fatigue syndrome (CFS) and long Covid.

The author's perspectives and ideas have helped her recover successfully from two periods of CFS and then from long Covid. Both conditions devastate the lives of the patients in our CFS Service. Ultimately, as clinicians we can only rule out treatable and significant disorders that could contribute to the four cardinal symptoms. These are debilitating fatigue after activity above an individual threshold which is much lower than expected; post-exertional malaise and symptom exacerbation; unrefreshing and often disturbed sleep; and cognitive dysfunction often called 'brain fog'.

We mainly focus on ruling out endocrine disorders and cancers. Often these conditions are diagnosed, and the patient can improve with respect to their symptoms and indeed have the benefit of a life improved in terms of morbidity and mortality. Overall, we only spend much less than an hour with our patients per year. Then they are discharged. Not ideal, but it is all we can deliver within an NHS service. But it is the other 8,759 hours the patient must live and manage on their own.

This book is a paradigm shift in treating CFS. It offers realistic and achievable changes in lifestyle and thinking that could lead to a life enhanced and renewed with considerably more energy. This book passionately entreats you, the person with CFS or long Covid, to make small positive changes.

I think ultimately the ideas outlined in the book have the potential to improve everyone's lives. There is ample evidence that attention to activity, rest, diet, spending time with nature, feeling gratitude, kindness to yourself, yoga, mindfulness and smiling can improve life – and reduce risk of chronic conditions such as diabetes, heart disease and even cancers.

As prescribing clinicians, we are very pleased when the 'fix' to a clinical problem is a drug. It often works. This book is as effective a therapy as any drug, and we can think of it in the same way as a drug such as a statin or an antidepressant. That is:

Therapeutic indication: Chronic fatigue syndrome (CFS), or long Covid
Mode of action: Helping you achieve hope towards recovery through gratitude, being kind to yourself, breathing techniques, smiling, time with nature, pacing, food and hydration advice, sleep restoration, beneficial habits, posture and yoga, good gut health and a holistic view of yourself.
Side effects: None. People may notice a more dynamic you and be disturbed!
Cost: None. Indeed, if not used, a life less lived well.

This book runs close to our clinic philosophy of asking patients to embrace the concept of *carpe diem* (seize the day). I will ensure that we have sufficient copies to give to some of our patients. We will certainly navigate the vast majority towards it.

This delightful fable with its intriguing metaphoric characters, with ample scientific credentials, can change your life! I hope you enjoy reading it and living it as much as I did and do.

Foreword

Professor Vinod Patel MD FRCP FHEA RCPath ME, MRCGP DRCOG MB ChB BSc (Hons)
Consultant in endocrinology and diabetes, acute medicine, chronic fatigue syndrome, Diabetes and Endocrinology Centre, George Eliot Hospital NHS Trust, Nuneaton, and professor of Diabetes and Clinical Skills, Warwick Medical School, University of Warwick

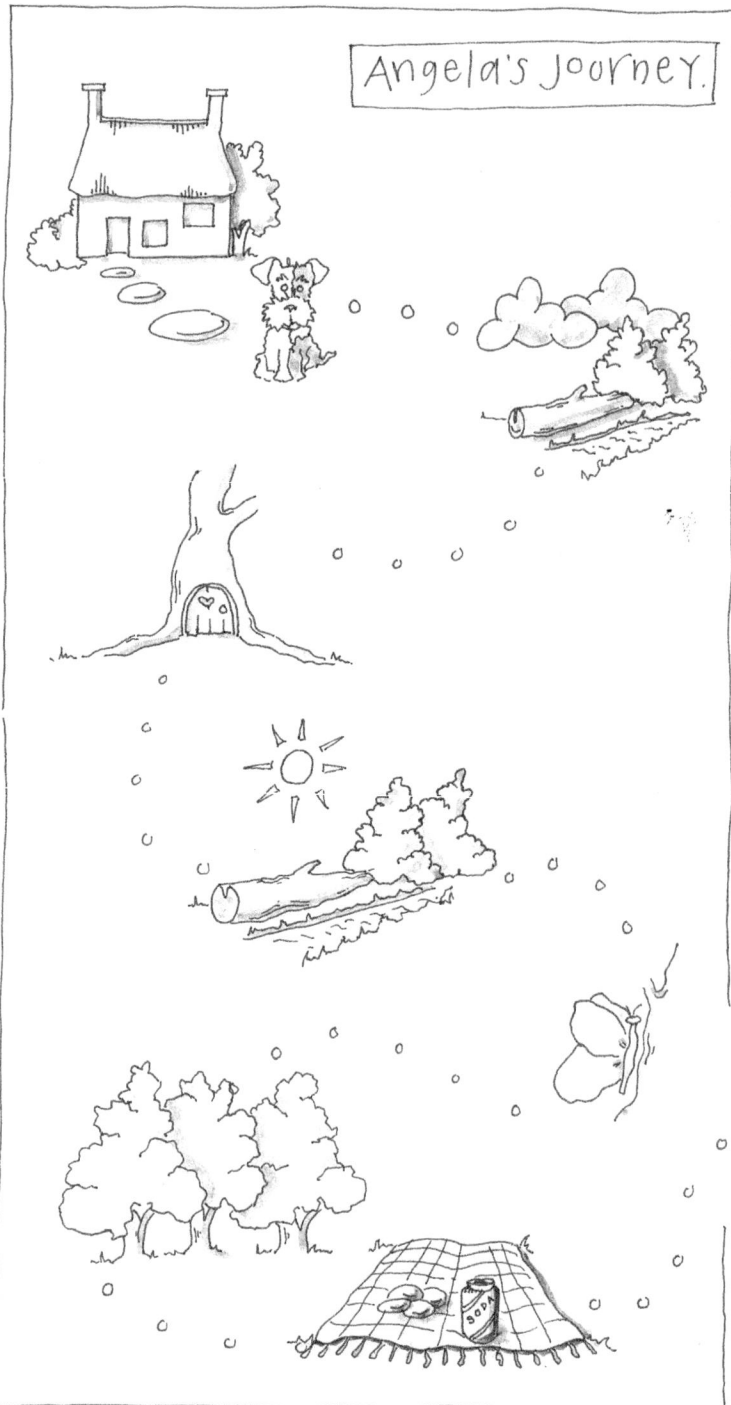

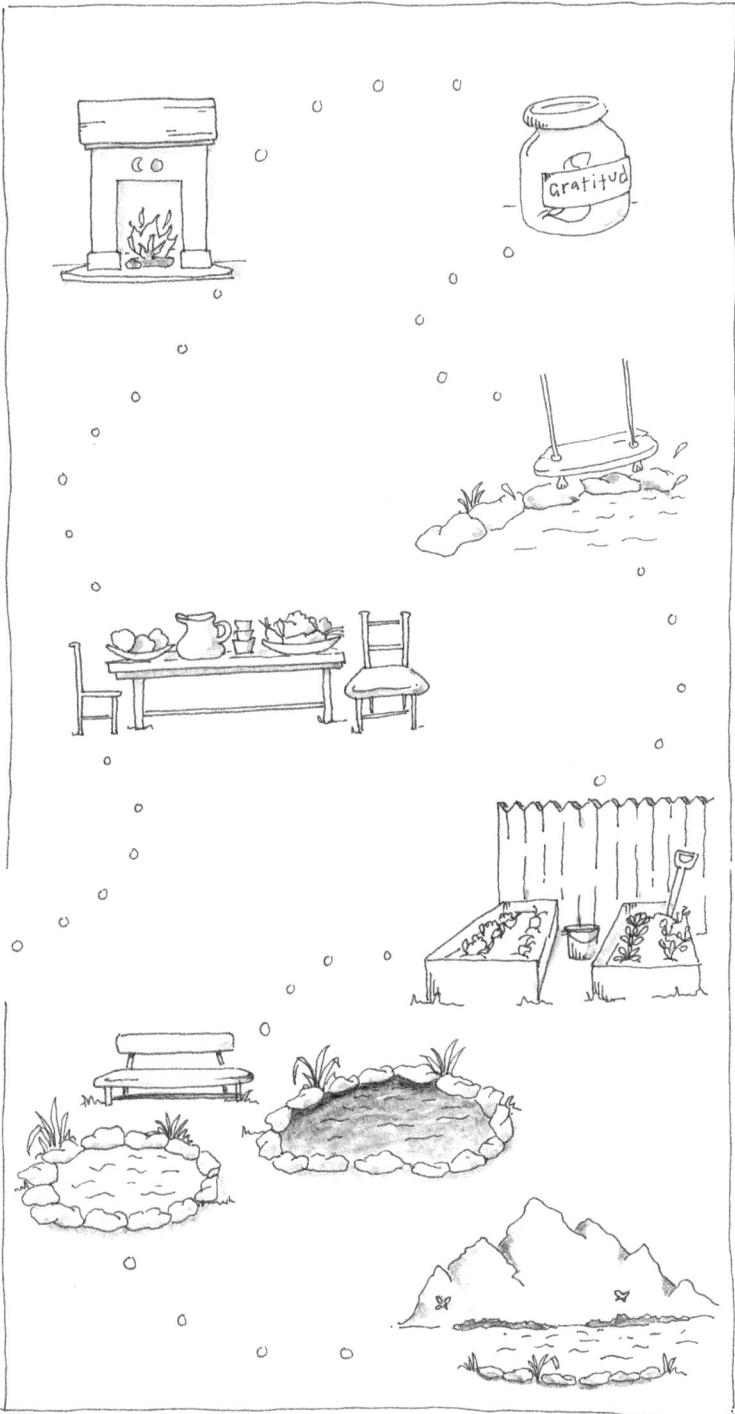

INTRODUCTION

Did you pick up this book because you're struggling with your energy levels? Would you like to know what you can do today to kick-start your recovery from long-term fatigue? When I was at the start of my journey with chronic fatigue syndrome (CFS) and later long Covid, when I didn't have the energy to do anything apart from lie in bed all day, I could have done with a book that was easy to understand, informative and didn't require a lot of effort to read. That's why I've written this book in a form of a story. It's light hearted, fun and magical – three things I desperately needed when I was in the throes of a living nightmare. A book like this would have saved me so much time and energy when I was searching for answers, so I hope it will save some for you.

I want you to know that there is hope. This book has it in abundance. I want to support you on your journey and share information that I've gathered and implemented over years of reading books and articles, attending courses and chronic fatigue clinics as well as helping others with their energy issues. You may have been diagnosed with long Covid, CFS – or as it's sometimes known, myalgic encephalomyelitis (ME). From now on, I'll be using the term CFS to cover both CFS and ME. This book is about energy – how to conserve it and how to lose it. More detailed information about CFS can be found in the resources section at the back of the book.

Before I go any further, let me explain why I understand what you're going through. I've had CFS twice, followed by long Covid. I feel as if I've been to hell and back several times. When I was first struggling with CFS, I lost who I was, as if my personality had been removed and replaced by someone I didn't know. I became sad, moody, quiet, reserved, angry and fed up. I lost my mojo and felt disconnected from everyone around me. I felt that life was unfair and didn't know if I'd ever get better. I was scared. Was this it? Was this going to be my life now, curled up in bed with no energy to do anything? It's a tough place to be. In fact, I'd go further than that and say I'd never want anyone to go through this. It's life changing and seemingly never ending. I felt as if I had no control over my body. CFS just seemed to take over and I was helpless to stop it. The days all seemed to merge and time stood still. For a while, I'd wake up every morning feeling the same. I hoped I'd feel some change, some improvement. Back then, I didn't understand why I had this condition – but I do now. If you have CFS, maybe you had a childhood illness such as glandular fever or suffered some kind of trauma. It's also connected to the state of your liver and gut, how many toxins you have in your body and whether you had food poisoning – the list goes on. There's more detail about this and the reasons why I had CFS in the resources section.

    The hardest part was trying to explain how I felt, because the only person who was experiencing it was me. I had no plaster, no bandage, nothing externally that I could show people. I only had my voice, my words to express my feelings and symptoms, which at times were complicated and varied from day to day. I wanted everyone to understand how I was feeling. I wanted to be believed but sadly that wasn't always the case. If only people could've felt what I was feeling just for one day, then they'd have experienced the overwhelming sense of helplessness when your body refuses to do what you want it to. Mine just wanted to lie down and rest. Is this resonating with you?

    CFS first hit me in 1993, when I was 27. It came

Introduction

completely out of the blue. I was working as a physiotherapist, playing sport, enjoying a great social life and doing a postgraduate course. I was newly married and very happy. In fact, life couldn't have been any better. I was the kind of person who never sat down; I was always on the go, driving myself to be better both physically and mentally. Pacing? What the hell was that? I didn't want to slow down. Then… CRASH. My life stopped overnight. I could hardly lift my head off the pillow. I had no energy to do anything. I managed to crawl into my local surgery and the GP just told me to go home and rest. They said I had a virus and it would go.

Even though I'd just got married, I moved back in with my parents. I couldn't get out of bed for months, apart from having a daily shower, which I found totally exhausting. That was my life. I had no idea what was going on and I was terrified. My symptoms were bizarre, including weakness down my left leg and brain fog. I was too tired to read and despite this overwhelming fatigue I couldn't sleep. I had headaches and zinging all over my body as if I'd put my hand into an electric socket. I had numerous blood tests and ended up having a brain scan to exclude any neurological condition such as multiple sclerosis (MS). Everything came back normal, which was frustrating because I wanted to understand what was happening to me; I wanted to be able to 'fix it'. I wanted to take a tablet and get better, but that didn't happen. My life came to a halt. I couldn't work. I couldn't play any sport. I couldn't socialise. I had no life – that had been taken away from me. I had no control.

After a few months, when everything else had been ruled out, my doctor came back with the diagnosis of CFS. In those days it was known as 'yuppie flu' and wasn't taken seriously. There was a stigma attached to it as if you were making it all up. That was so infuriating – I wanted to shout at people and ask them to swap places. I was told to keep resting and take it easy. I stayed with my parents for a few months. Luckily my mum was a good cook and a positive person, which made a huge difference. She was my rock. My dad was around too but Mum was there for me every step of the way. My husband came to see me at weekends and was a huge support but more importantly he believed everything I told him about how I felt. I didn't have to convince him. Others, yes, but never him. Thinking about it now, it must have been so hard for the people around me who were trying to help and support me because they felt helpless as well.

After a few months I was able to go downstairs and even managed a short walk around the garden. That was a huge milestone and I still remember today how I felt. Small steps are to be celebrated when you feel that rough. I did begin to feel better over time but had absolutely no idea how to help myself at the start, apart from resting. I was given no guidance at all. I went back to live with my husband and started doing short walks, building them up gradually. I felt like a snail, so different to the athlete I was before this happened. It was a slow and hard journey. Friends were kind but didn't understand what I was going through. The only thing I remember doing, which was recommended by a friend, was to see a kinesiologist. She was wonderful and helped me feel as if I had some control. At last, I was given some guidance about what I could do for myself. Using muscle-testing techniques, she helped me to look at foods that might have been aggravating my symptoms. When you've felt out of control for so long it's a massive deal. Being told there was something I could do other than rest was a huge step forward in my recovery.

I did return to work part time but it took years before I felt fully myself again. Back then it was just a matter of being patient, giving in to all the signs and symptoms and resting when I needed to. It felt like a long, long journey with many struggles along the way – ups and downs and crashes and frustrations. It's often a multifaceted condition, affecting many different organs and systems in the body. Are you still with me? Is this making sense to you? It's a complex, debilitating condition.

My second episode of CFS was in 2016, when I was 50. Again, I was working as a physiotherapist, playing sport and having a great social life but I'd just lost my mum, to whom I was very close. I was absolutely devastated. She was taken too young and too quickly. I'd also moved house and had major surgery... CRASH. This time I knew what was going on but it didn't change how I felt. Like before, I was angry, frustrated, fed up, emotional, sad. I was back on the sofa, unable to work or go out. My symptoms were similar but not quite as extreme. My eye muscles were struggling and I couldn't read, so I became reliant on the radio, podcasts and audiobooks. I went to my GP, who advised me to rest (again). It was incredibly frustrating but eventually the GP referred me to the NHS chronic fatigue clinic at the George Eliot Hospital NHS Trust. There was a long waiting list but I eventually got an appointment and it helped me to understand the importance of pacing myself. That proved to be crucial to my recovery.

Having to say no to fun things, no to seeing friends and not being able to work or play sport was heartbreaking. I felt very alone. In fact, for a while, I cut myself off from the outside world. I didn't want to know how much fun everyone else was having. I wasn't in a good place mentally or physically but I was lucky to have the support of my amazing family – my husband and children (Georgie and Nick). But I felt guilty that I'd become so reliant on them to do everything. This is hard to do if it's not in your nature to ask for help. I was much better at giving help; I wasn't so good at receiving it. Gradually, I began to accept help from other family members and friends and once I'd let them in, they were amazing. For instance, a lovely group of local friends did my gardening because they knew how important it was to me. Others came and sat at the end of the sofa for a chat or delivered food parcels for the family. I'm grateful to each one of them for their kindness and support.

My recovery journey really started when I saw a nutritionist locally and then went on a nutritional healing course with the Nutritional Healing Foundation. The thought of going on a course seemed far fetched at the time but I decided to see if I could manage it. I warned the organisers that I might not be able to cope. They were understanding and supportive on my first day and throughout the course. It was life changing. I felt I had regained some control over my life and was given some amazing tools to try. The main change I made for the first four months was to increase my water consumption. I bought a water filter and was drinking up to four pints a day. I carried on with the course and it taught me so much. I eventually qualified as a naturopathic nutritionist and ended up being a homework marker for other students on the course.

After the focus on keeping hydrated, I started to make other changes to my diet. I began to turn a corner. I slowly implemented all that I had learned on the course but made other changes too. I started some gentle yoga and began to walk in the countryside. As my energy improved, I wanted to know what else I could do. I was determined to find out as much as I could. I completed courses on psychology, meditation, yoga, Pilates, gut health, mindfulness – the list goes on. The Optimal Health Clinic (OHC) was extremely helpful at this stage and I consulted with a nutritionist and completed meditation and psychology programmes there.

My recovery journey was up and down and all over the place. I pushed, then I crashed. I picked myself up and tried again. It was tough and excruciatingly frustrating at times. When I look back at my journal it reminds me that I had some dark days. But I was determined not to give up and continued to implement many new techniques.

Introduction

The latter stage of my recovery was about focusing on my mindset and the mind–body connection. At times this was way out of my comfort zone but it was key to my recovery.

    I can't believe I'm writing this, but in a strange and astonishing way, I'm grateful to have had CFS because I've been on an epic journey of self-discovery that I would never have embarked on otherwise. I now have powerful tools that will help me for the rest of my life and for that I'm grateful. I never thought in a million years that I'd be admitting that. My recovery has taken me on many journeys – I've learned how to put a plastic straw through a potato, how to make sauerkraut, how to nostril breathe, how to love myself and my cells, how to laugh at my mistakes, how to meditate, how to eat food that benefits your gut health and how to use the Emotional Freedom Technique (EFT) to reduce stress and anxiety.

    I also learned how to acknowledge old beliefs but not let them have power, how to reach my higher self, how to pace myself, how to ask for help, the key supplements and nutrition I need, the importance of having a good bowel movement every day and how to care for my liver. Hopefully you get the picture.

    Over the next few years, I began to feel so much better and was doing well. But then, CRASH... I was hit with Covid and it went on for months. I was back in bed, struggling with my breathing and feeling absolutely rubbish. I couldn't believe that I was back here again. This time, though, my mindset was different and that really helped me to cope and stay positive. As before, my social life stopped and so did my work and sport. Covid is another complex condition that can affect many systems in the body but all the knowledge I'd gathered over the years helped enormously. I was able to rest well and managed to avoid being admitted to hospital, mainly due to the breathing techniques I'd learned. It's scary when your breathing is affected and I had to calm myself down when

I could feel the fear rising. I recovered but it took time and sheer determination. It was a roller coaster ride and even though I knew about pacing, I didn't always stick to it. I overdid it and ended up back on the sofa a few times.

I'm pleased to report that I'm now back at the gym and have even returned to rowing. I also have a great social life and my own business, which allows me to bring all my knowledge together as a physiotherapist, acupuncturist, lecturer and naturopathic nutritionist with a wealth of knowledge in many other areas, especially involving mindset. I've learned to listen to my body and what it needs and understand that if I ignore it, I'll pay the price! I don't have all the solutions; I'm not at the end of my journey and it has taken me a long time to understand what makes a difference with CFS. If you want to continue following my journey you can join me on my Instagram account @nutrition2energise.

Everyone's signs and symptoms are slightly different but the similarity is an overwhelming feeling of fatigue. Think of the body as comprised of units of energy. We only have so much energy in each second, minute, hour, day, week, month, etc. I found that how I used that energy was crucial to my recovery whether it was in relation to the food I ate, to my mindset, to whom I spoke, keeping to a baseline or not pushing too hard too soon. Once I had this concept of units of energy in my head, I thought, 'How can I put this across to all ages in a way that everyone will understand and relate to?'

My intention in writing this book is to share my toolbox for managing energy in the form of a fable. My protagonist is called Angela. Each chapter follows Angela's journey and who she meets along the way to help and guide her (beautifully illustrated by Lynn Redwood). There's a summary of key points at the end of each chapter to help clarify what has been covered. If you'd like to know more, the resources section at the end of the book expands on

Introduction

what has happened in each chapter and the theory behind the tools.

Angela enters a magical world where she's given marbles of energy. As she continues her journey, she learns about what she can do to maintain or gain energy and what will rob her of energy. With every character she meets, she discovers a little more about how to use her energy wisely. She has a mission to achieve and needs to stay focused on this. Her mission is to reach the Butterfly Mountain, which stands by a lake. Why, you may ask, a butterfly mountain? I came up with the idea of comparing the journey of recovery to the life cycle of a butterfly. There are four stages:

1. The eggs are laid on a leaf.
2. They hatch into caterpillars, which feed on the leaf.
3. They hang upside down to form a chrysalis.
4. The butterfly emerges, lays more eggs, and the cycle continues.

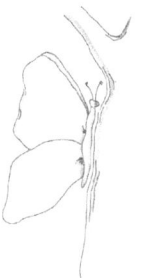

Where are you in the life cycle of CFS? Are you at the beginning of your journey or coming out the other end and

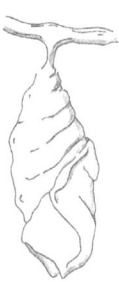

emerging as a butterfly? It doesn't really matter where you are in the cycle; what's important is that the choices you make today can impact your future. The eggs are the beginning of your journey with CFS – your signs and symptoms. The leaf represents the foundations – the brilliant choices that you make or have made up until now. You want to be feeding off those brilliant choices and doing the basics well. The ideas I'm going to share through Angela's journey are your nourishment, your fuel. The caterpillar is you as you grow and learn – moving around on the leaf and feeding off your knowledge so that you can grow stronger. Then comes the chrysalis stage. This is about you giving yourself time to implement these ideas and look after yourself. Immerse yourself in your healing – if you want to hang upside down then feel free! Because the only person who can totally look after you is *you*. Your body knows what you need – use your intuition and listen to what it's telling you. Be kind to yourself. If you're out of sync with your body and mind, you'll struggle. The butterfly is you emerging from CFS/long Covid as a new person with fresh knowledge and self-belief.

Are you ready? Then let's meet Angela, who will narrate her own story.

CHAPTER 1

HUGO HOPE AND THE MAGIC MARBLES OF ENERGY

Fight or flight and rest and repair

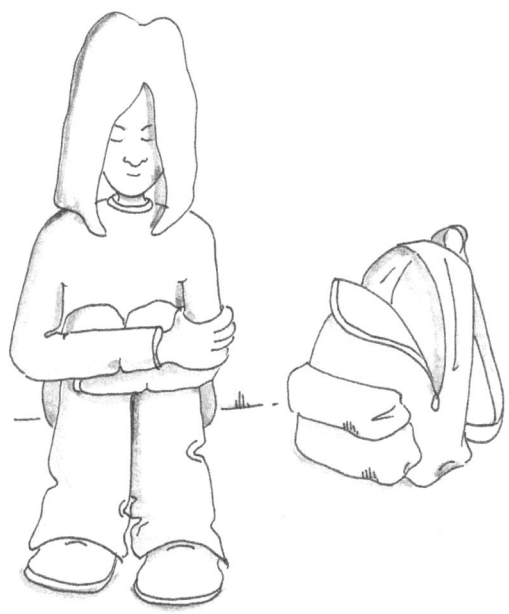

'All my tests have come back normal,' I confirm to the GP. 'So what's the diagnosis?'

'The only possibility that remains,' the GP replies, 'is that you have chronic fatigue syndrome, or

CFS. Everyone has a different presentation but the main symptom is overwhelming fatigue, which is what you've been suffering from the most.'

'So what's the treatment?'

'You just have to take it easy, rest and see what happens.'

'Is that it?'

'Yes,' says the GP.

And that's it. The phone goes dead. I let it fall from my hand onto the rug I'm standing on. 'Well, that's rubbish,' I think to myself. I slump down into the green armchair behind me, put my head in my hands and sigh. The springs in the armchair are going, which means I can sink down into it. The old velvet arms are soft and feel as if they're embracing me. Despite how knackered and stained it is, it's my favourite chair. It has been through a lot with me. It's my go-to chair when I feel down. It feels like a cocoon.

So I have a diagnosis but no treatment. What on earth am I supposed to do now? I feel completely devastated. To be told I have CFS and must put up with it is utterly demoralising. I've had the rug pulled from under me. I feel I have no control over my life. I feel disempowered. I've been told there's nothing I can do but rest. Nothing! I used to have a life but I don't have one now. I'm barely surviving. In fact, I'm barely existing. You probably want to know all 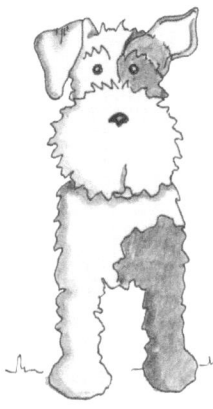 about me but I don't feel like going into that right now. Anyway, who'd want to know about Angela, the 30-year-old woman who lives on her own in a little thatched cottage? I'm not very interesting or fun. I used to be. Oh yes, I did; I was the life and soul of any party. Boy oh boy, could I party! I also used to have a great job, play tennis, row and have a great social life. I can't manage to do any of those things now. I do at least have a gorgeous 10-year-old dog called Lexi.

The phone rings. I reach down to pick it up. It's Catherine again. I don't answer. I know she means well and is just checking up on me but I can't be bothered to talk to her right now. I can't be bothered to talk to anyone right now. It's too exhausting and I don't want to hear about the great night out she had, dancing and having fun. Why would I? Those unkind thoughts are so unlike me! This FCS or whatever it's called hasn't just taken all my energy – I feel as if I've changed personalities and lost the person I was. I'm not sure I like this different me at all but I just can't seem to stop myself having negative, unhelpful thoughts.

I decide the best thing to do is take Lexi for a walk. I'm just about to climb the rickety old staircase to get changed when I catch a glimpse of myself in the mirror. God, I look awful! My hair is lank and hangs limply around my pale, drawn face. I have bags under my eyes from lack of sleep, despite the fact that all I want to do is sleep. Is that really me? I used to take pride in my appearance. I had lovely glowing skin and sparkling eyes. Where have I gone? I know I'm in there somewhere; I just need to get me back. As I climb the stairs, I look outside at the neglected garden and its weeds. Even my garden looks dejected.

I grab my phone and put my usual bits and pieces in a rucksack – iPod, dog treats, poo bags, a few snacks and a drink. Lexi's lead goes on next and we set off. It isn't raining but it feels as if a storm is brewing. The clouds are dark and menacing. Thank goodness I've bought a raincoat just in case. I follow my usual meandering path onto the hills behind the cottage. It's a strange sort of day today. I can't quite put my finger on it but things don't seem quite 'normal'. It feels as if I'm looking at everything through a pair of brightly coloured spectacles. I shake it off and after a while sit down on a log, which is a bit damp and covered in moss. It's been raining so the stream is quite high and running fast. I sit and watch as it runs over and around the rocks and pebbles.

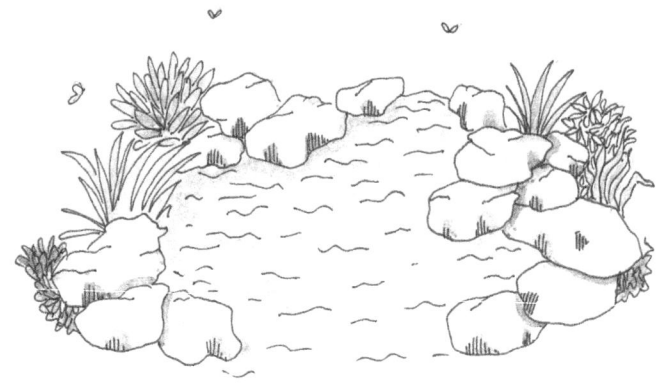

I've been to this spot many times before but each time it feels different. Lexi also loves this spot and is jumping around in the stream with sheer joy, her tail wagging madly. I just sit and connect with my surroundings – the sound of the stream, the ominous clouds, the smell of the pine trees, the feel of the soft moss under my fingertips. I also connect with my thoughts, which aren't great today. I'm feeling low and frustrated after my conversation with the GP. I feel the log move and look up. It's Catherine. Surely she can read my body language? I don't want anyone else near me. She just looks and me and says, 'I knew you'd be at your favourite spot. I know you're struggling but I'm always here for you. Anyway, I've come to return your front door key – I borrowed it the other day.'

I thank her, taking the key, and at that moment a huge wave of fatigue hits me, so I close my eyes for a while and feel the key in my hands. As I drift off, I imagine it becoming a beautiful, ornate key and start to wonder what it might open. In my dreamlike state, I get up and feel drawn to a magnificent oak tree nearby. I can see a small door with a keyhole in the bark. It's not obvious but it's there.

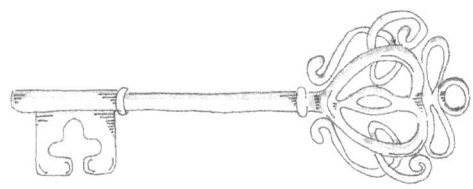

'How amazing,' I think to myself. 'I pass this tree most days and I've never noticed the door before.' I start to wonder if the beautiful key will unlock this door. I gingerly put the key into the lock. It fits and I begin to turn it. I gently push open the door and peer through it. I can see a wood on the other side, a mirror image of the one I'm standing in. I decide to step through the door.

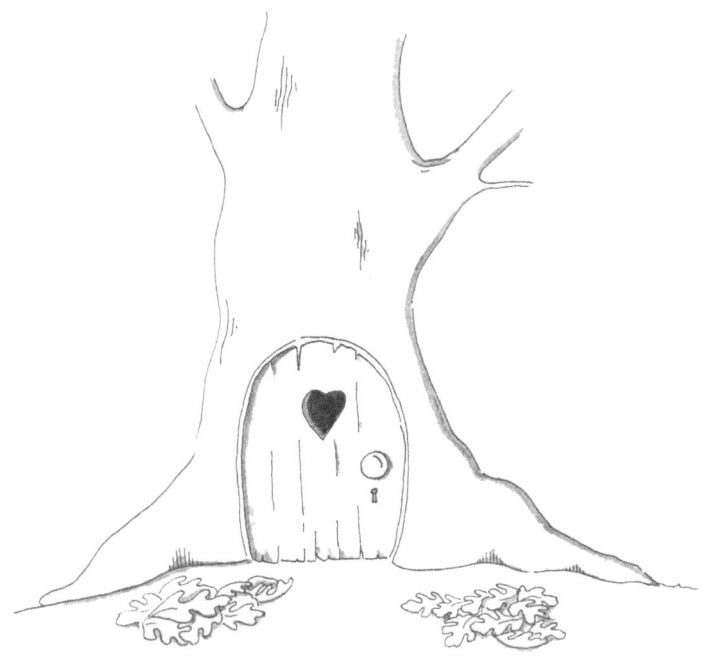

The opening is quite small, so I must do a bit of manoeuvring to get myself through. Lexi just bounces in. Even the menacing clouds look the same and I can see the log that Catherine and I were just sitting on. But there's no Catherine. Instead there's a gentleman there. He has a lovely warm, welcoming smile and is beckoning me to come over and sit with him. He's wearing a waistcoat and a black bowler hat and is carrying a black cane. Embedded in the cane's handle is a butterfly. He looks completely out of place, especially with his black patent shoes, which don't even look muddy.

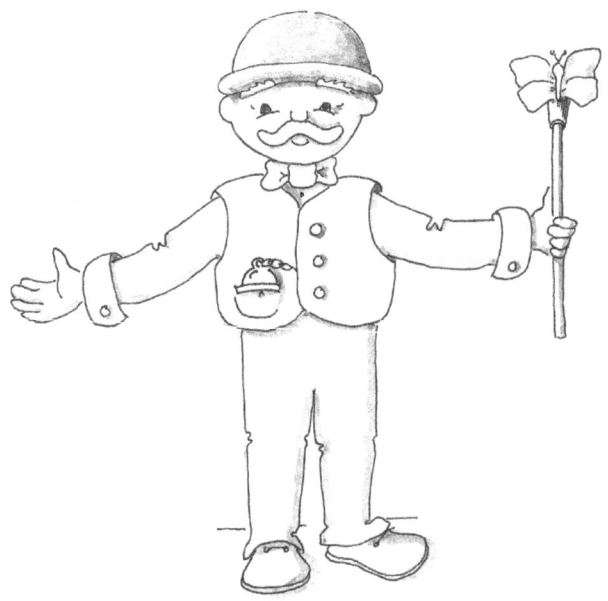

He smiles at me and introduces himself as Hugo Hope. He reminds me of a character called Mr Benn that I used to watch on TV as a young girl. He goes on to say, 'You're going to go on a journey – a long journey to the magical Butterfly Mountain, which stands next to a beautiful lake. I have a mission for you. This mission will help you to find some of the answers you're looking for. It will help to give you some ideas about how you can start to help yourself.'

I look at him in complete shock. What on earth is he talking about? I rub my eyes, look again but he's still there. He takes out of his pocket a beautiful embroidered black velvet bag with gold string around the top. He loosens the string, opens the bag and pours the contents into his hand. Ten marbles fall out and I can't take my eyes off them. Each one of the marbles is small, perfectly round and smooth, and appears to have all the colours of the rainbow inside it. And it looks as if the colours are swirling around. I'm mesmerised by these marbles. Then Hugo puts them into my hands. I can feel their smooth texture as I roll them around. They feel powerful and strong.

'These marbles are magical,' he says. 'Each marble represents a unit of energy. Energy is essential to all living organisms and plays a major part in helping you recover. I want you to take all ten marbles to the Butterfly Mountain. But you must understand that when you go on your journey, if you engage in activities that put you into the fight or flight response you'll lose marbles – but you'll gain them by putting yourself into the rest and repair 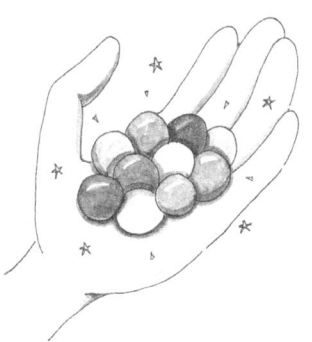 response. When this happens, the marbles will disappear from or appear in your hand. If you stay too long in the fight or flight response, you'll lose all the marbles and won't be able to complete the mission as you'll have used up all your energy. And please remember a very important point – you can't be in both responses at the same time.'

I'm wondering why I should take on this mission but realise I have nothing to lose. My life can't get any worse. If there's a small chance of improving it, why wouldn't I give it a go? But I need to ask Hugo Hope a question.

'So how do I know when I'm in the fight and fight response or the rest and repair one?'

'When you're in the fight or flight response your body is reacting to danger or stress,' Hugo explains. 'If you need to, let's say, avoid an approaching vehicle, it gives your body a burst of energy. You'll feel an increase in heart rate and blood pressure that will make you feel tense and on edge. In this state your body is in survival mode, so other functions such as digestion are put on the back burner. Sometimes people get stuck in this response due to such things as chronic stress, which can cause havoc in the body. In the rest and repair response the body is relaxed and conserves energy so that key functions such as digestion and repair can take place. That's why it's also called the rest and digest response. When you're in rest and repair your heart rate and breathing rate will slow down. It also helps to stimulate digestion and allows the body to enter the healing state, which is what you want.

'You'll learn more along the way about these two responses. That's why this mission is so important to you. If you manage to take all ten marbles to the Butterfly Mountain, you'll find your reward. Never lose focus on your mission. Where your focus goes, your energy will flow. Just use your intuition. Don't worry about how you'll get there; just stay focused on reaching the next objective. Now, close your eyes.'

He puts his hand on the side of my head and the Butterfly Mountain and the lake appear in my mind's eye. It's so beautiful. The sun is shining, the sky is clear blue and the Butterfly Mountain is reflected in the lake. There are butterflies of all different colours and sizes flying through the air. I feel my heart sing with joy. It's so peaceful and tranquil here that I can't help but smile to myself. The water looks so inviting that I can see myself putting my hand in and feeling it flow over my fingertips. Hugo asks me to open my eyes and hands me the butterfly that's embedded in the top of his cane. He tells me to keep this with me as I go on my journey. 'It's a symbol to remind you of your mission,' he says. 'It will help to keep you focused but it's also a symbol of hope, of never giving up regardless of how steep the path to recovery might be.' I take it from him with thanks and put it into my rucksack.

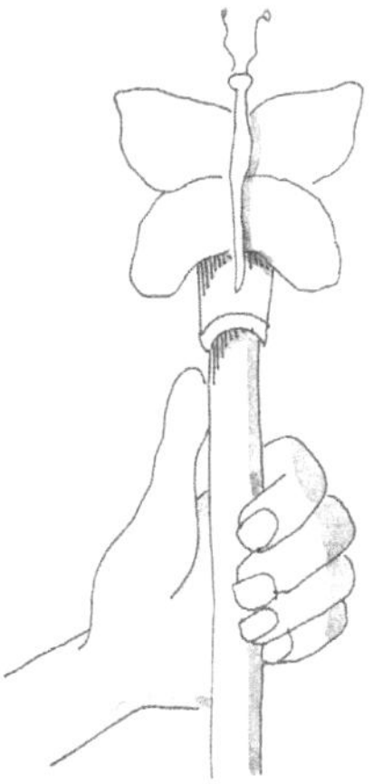

'There will be signs along the way that will show you which way to go,' he says. 'They will all be in the shape of a butterfly and attached to trees or fence posts.'

I feel the need to check everything he's just told me. 'To be clear, I'm going on a long journey to a magic Butterfly Mountain. There will be butterfly signs along the way pointing in the direction I need to take. To receive my reward I must have all ten magic marbles with me when I reach the mountain. Each marble is a unit of energy and I can gain or lose marbles depending on whether I'm in the fight or flight response or the rest and repair one – but I can't be in both states at the same time.'

'Yes,' says Hugo Hope. 'That sums it up perfectly. Good luck and remember to keep focused on what you want, which is to reach the magic Butterfly Mountain with all ten marbles. Where your focus goes, your energy will flow.'

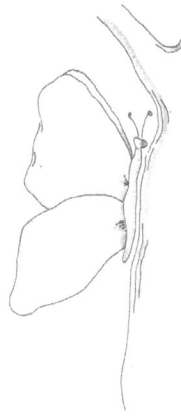

He points to a yellow butterfly on the tree in front of us, with an arrow pointing straight ahead. He wishes me luck, hands me a card then quietly walks away and seems to vanish into thin air. I'm speechless. I look at the card, which says:

Always have hope.
Stay in the rest and repair state.
Where your focus goes, your energy will flow.

I open my hands and look at the marbles. They're beautiful, hypnotic and feel powerful. But when I think about what I've been asked to do, I feel terrified! I can feel myself start to panic about whether I can complete this task. How am I going to find the signs? Will they be obvious? What happens if I don't get all ten marbles to the mountain? Will I know when I'm in these responses? My mind is racing. I can feel my heart rate and breathing rate increase, my hands feel clammy and I'm beginning to sweat.

I look down at the marbles and realise that I only have eight. I'm confused; why have I already lost two marbles? I must have put myself into the fight or flight response through my own thoughts. How am I going to get out of this? Hugo Hope talked about rest and repair so I need to think of a way that will bring down my heart rate and slow my breathing. I look at the marbles again and see the colours swirling around and I'm sure I can see the Butterfly Mountain in them. I let my mind drift to the mountain and the lake. I can see the butterflies, smell the flowers on the banks of the lake and see the ripples on the water. I can taste the water as well – it's fresh and tastes divine, so pure and clean. I can see myself taking a sip from the lake. The water feels so smooth and silky against my skin and throat.

I feel a sense of calm drift over me and notice that my heart rate has gone down and the clammy feeling has gone. I look at the marbles. All ten are back in my hand – and I've put them there through the power of my imagination. I've been able to bring myself out of the fight or flight response and into the rest and repair state. With Lexi by my side,

I leave the log behind and set off, following the yellow butterfly sign that I've just spotted here.

Key points

- To aid recovery, your body needs to be in the rest and repair response.
- The fight or flight response puts your body under stress, so you don't want to stay in it for too long.
- Your thoughts alone can put you into the fight or flight response or take you out of it into the rest and repair response.
- You can't be in both responses at the same time.
- Where your focus goes, your energy flows.
- Energy is essential to all living organisms and is the key to recovery, so learn how to use it wisely.

CHAPTER 2

BARBARA BELLOWS, BILLIE BUBBLE AND HENRY HAPPY

Breathwork, a protective bubble and the importance of smiling

I look back and the door in the oak tree seems to have vanished. This is like a parallel universe. Everything seems the same but I know it's different. I need to keep my focus on where I'm going because I want the reward. I like a challenge – I always have. I'm a great starter but not always a finisher, so this mission will be tough. The yellow butterfly sign is pointing straight ahead, so off I go with Lexi by my side, following the path through the pine and oak trees. I have no idea how long this journey is going to take so I pull out my iPod and decide to listen to an audiobook. Despite being in this surreal place, I'm still struggling with being told I have CFS, so I think I'll listen to something that reflects my mood. Why not a horror story? That's what I feel I'm in: a horror story that ends in doom and gloom.

I find an appropriate one called *The Mist*. I feel as if I'm in a mist or fog and can't seem to find a way out, so it fits perfectly. I press play as Lexi runs by my side. I become totally immersed in this scary story. The oak trees seem to be grabbing at me with their long, interwoven branches and every sound seems to be twice as loud as normal. Suddenly a twig snaps behind me and I scream and jump a mile. My heart is pounding and I'm breathing heavily. I swing round and see Lexi bounding away. I can feel myself give a big sigh of relief but I can't switch off the audiobook. I need to know whether the characters survive. I feel the fear continue to rise inside me. It feels as if the oxygen is being sucked out of the air around me. A sudden scream from above makes me jump back and stare up into the canopy of trees. My heart is racing even faster and then I see a bird of prey. It looks like a kite, with a distinctive fork in its tail. My heart is about to leap out through my chest. I stop and try to calm myself. I turn off the audiobook and look around. I put my hand in my pocket and feel for the marbles. I roll them around in my fingers and notice that I only have six. How on earth have I lost four marbles? Then I remember what Hugo Hope told me. He said that I will lose a marble if I put myself into the fight or flight response, which is what I must be doing now. OK, so I need to get myself into the rest and repair response. I sit down on a nearby log to stop and think.

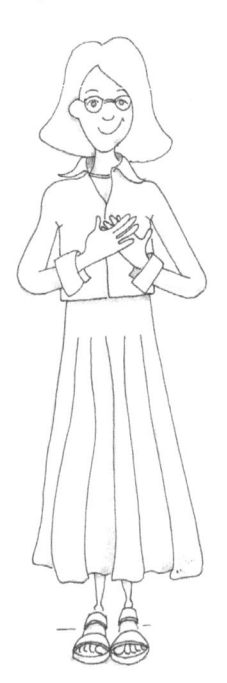

Then I hear someone coming. I don't want to be interrupted today. I want to be with my own thoughts. I'm about to turn my back on whoever it is that's encroaching on my space when I see a woman approaching with her hands placed against her chest. I see beside her a black cane and on the top is a beautiful, tiny pair of bellows. She introduces herself as Barbara Bellows, a breathwork teacher.

'Are you OK? You look very shaken,' she says.

'Oh, I've just been listening to a horror story and was scared out of my wits,' I explain. 'And now I've lost four of my magic marbles! I need to get them back. Can you help?'

'I find breathing techniques really help me when I start to panic or feel scared,' she answers. 'I find them calming, they refocus my mind and I can centre myself again. They help me to put myself into a lovely rest and repair state.'

'Would you mind showing me?'

I watch Barbara as she sits up straight, closes her eyes and puts one hand on her belly and the other on her chest. She then counts to four as she breathes in, seven as she holds her breath and then breathes out through pursed lips for a count of eight. She repeats this a couple of times and then opens her eyes. She suggests I should try it. I can feel the air flood into my lungs and my belly pulls away from my right hand as I breathe out. I do this four times and feel an overwhelming sense of calm and tranquillity. I slowly open my eyes and see that Barbara is smiling. She goes on to tell me about some other breathing techniques. For instance, just breathing in for four then breathing out for six through pursed lips.

'You can do this for ten minutes in the morning and evening or whenever you need to calm yourself,' she says. Then she takes the pair of bellows from the top of her cane and hands it to me. 'This will remind you about the importance of breathwork to calm and centre yourself and put yourself back into the rest and repair response.' She hands me a card, points to a tree that has a green butterfly on it and slowly walks away.

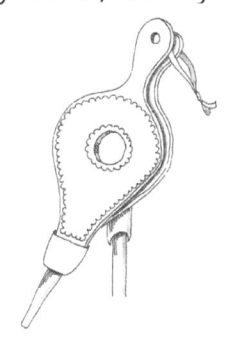

I look at the card. There's a quote on it from the spiritual teacher Thich Nhat Hanh:

**Breathing in, I calm my body. Breathing out, I smile.
Dwelling in the present moment,
I know this is the only moment.**

I feel for the marbles and all ten have been restored. I never would've thought that breathing techniques could help to restore my sense of calm, put me in a restful state and help me reconnect with myself. Well, that's how I feel right now. I put the bellows and card into my rucksack and follow the green butterfly sign on the tree.

'Right, Angela,' I say to myself. 'Keep focused, don't get distracted – magic Butterfly Mountain, here I come!' I get my iPod out again. I need to listen to something inspiring, something that will help me to stay focused and determined.

I find an audiobook that had been recommended to me about an inspirational woman called Edith Eger, who wrote a book called *The Choice* (2018). It's a story about hope, inspiration and humanity. It's based on Edith's life – she survived the Auschwitz concentration camp as a child and then became an eminent psychologist. It's thought provoking and at times tough to listen to but such a moving and inspirational story about survival in unbelievable circumstances. What an impressive woman she is. Edith is so powerful with her thoughts – she's always positive and never gives up. One paragraph really resonates with me: 'No one can make you a victim but you. We become victims not because of what happens to us but when we choose to hold onto our victimisation. We develop a victim's mind – a way of thinking and being that is rigid, stuck in the past, pessimistic, blaming, unforgiving. We become our own jailor when we choose the confines of the victim's mind.'

Is that what I'm doing right now? Behaving like a victim, as if I have no choices or options? I certainly feel pessimistic and stuck about the diagnosis of CFS. My jailor is CFS – or maybe it's also my mindset? Maybe I'm saying all the wrong things to myself. Why can't I just be given a tablet that will make me feel better? Just because Edith has overcome extreme pain and adversity to lead a fulfilling life doesn't mean that I will. 'Come on, Angela,' I say to myself. 'That's so unhelpful.'

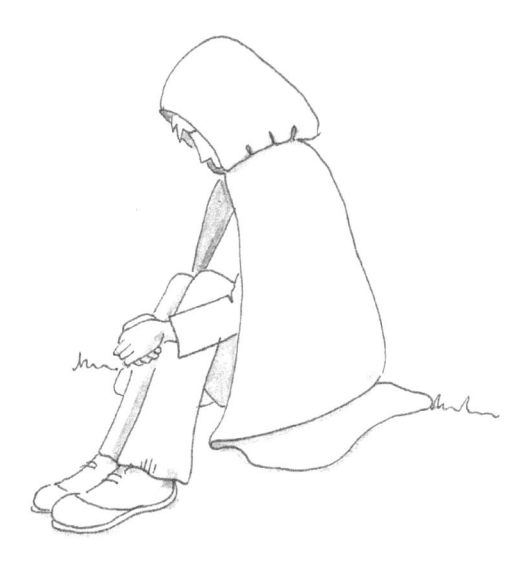

As I continue to walk and listen, I become aware of someone sitting just ahead of me. They are hunched over, wearing a black cape with the hood up. I stop the audiobook to ask if they're OK. They stand up, walk with me and start to speak in a quiet voice about how awful their life is. They talk about their home life, their relationships and their job. I listen intently and feel myself getting caught up in their story. My whole focus is now on them. I begin to feel their pain, anxiety and frustration. It feels as if I'm falling under their spell. As I'm listening, I put my hand in my pocket and start to roll the marbles around with my fingers. I start to count and notice that I only have six marbles left again. That doesn't make sense to me. How can I lose four marbles just by listening to somebody? The person stops, stands up straight and takes down their hood. They have short-cropped black hair and are about the same age as me. It's only then that I notice they're holding a black cane topped by a golden ball.

They look me straight in the eye and say, 'We've been walking for quite a while now and you've listened carefully to all my negativity, asking what you can do to help me.

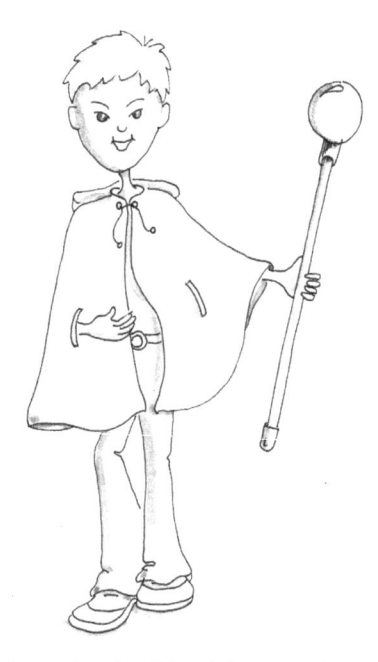

You're obviously a natural helper but I've taken a lot of your energy; I've drained you with my negative thoughts, which is why you've lost four marbles. I'm going to suggest a way of protecting yourself in the future so you can set your boundaries and not let other people's thoughts and emotions affect you. I want you to close your eyes and visualise a beautiful golden bubble surrounding and protecting you. You feel safe in this bubble, as if nothing can get through. You can breathe inside this bubble and remain calm and centred. Then I want you to visualise words and letters bouncing off this bubble as if you're wearing a massive inflatable sumo wrestling suit. That's the power of this bubble. I want you to feel it. But remember that the bubble isn't fixed; it's ever changing and evolving. Think of a soap bubble – it can be burst by you or others but remember that you can recreate it. You can create a new bubble around you, maybe in a different colour.'

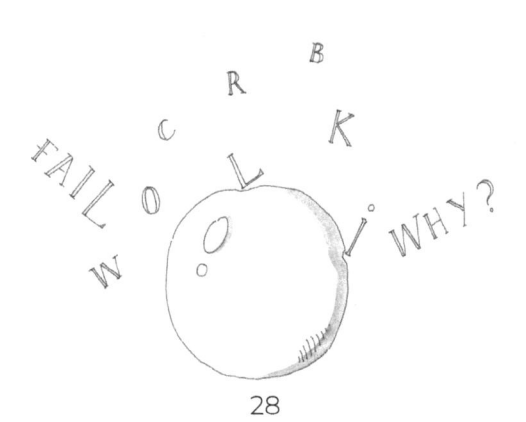

I begin to visualise a beautiful golden bubble all around me, protecting me and not letting other people's unhelpful words enter. I put my hand back in my pocket and feel eight marbles. I've regained two, which feels great. When I open my eyes the person introduces themselves as Billie Bubble, a therapist. Billie proceeds to give me the golden bubble from the top of their cane.

'This is to remind you to protect yourself from other people's unhelpful words that would otherwise drain you of energy. The golden ball also represents your environment, what and who you surround yourself with, including what you listen to. Your body doesn't know the difference between whether you're scared because of what you've been listening to or scared because you're in danger and need to run for your life. Both situations will put you into the fight or flight response. Make sure that what you're listening to is positive, helpful and uplifting. Then you'll start to believe that recovery is possible. You're in control of your environment 24 hours a day so use that time wisely.'

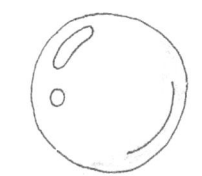

Billie points to a golden butterfly sign attached to a fence post that points straight ahead and gives me a card. Written on it are the words:

**Before starting your day, take a moment
to imagine a golden bubble around your body.
Invite people in or keep them out.
Be aware of your environment.**

I put the golden ball and card into my rucksack with the other symbols I've collected. I call Lexi and set off again. Just as my mind is drifting off, thinking about the fact that I'm still two marbles down, I notice a man coming towards me, smiling and singing as if he doesn't have a care in the world. As we get closer together, I can hear him singing one of my favourite Beatles songs, 'Twist and Shout'. He's also holding a black cane and on the top is a silver smile. He's twizzling it around in his hands, throwing it up then catching it again. His positive energy is contagious. I can feel a smile spread across my face as I watch him enjoying himself. Joy seems to be filling my whole body. This smiling person introduces himself as Henry Happy, grabs me by the arm and starts swinging me around. He starts singing again and I start singing too! I haven't sung like this for ages and it feels good. I start thinking of the movie I associate the song with – *Ferris Bueller's Day Off*. I haven't thought about this film for years! As the song finishes, we both smile and laugh.

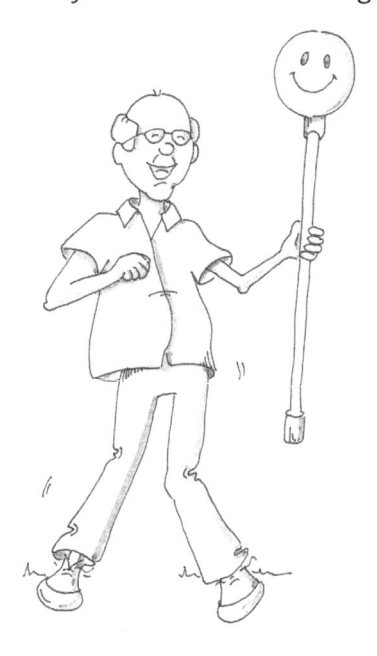

He takes the silver smile off the top of his cane, hands it to me and tells me that smiling can release feel-good hormones such as serotonin and endorphins, which help to put your body into the rest and repair response (he also explains that serotonin acts as a neurotransmitter). He gives me a card, which I read out loud:

**Never forget the power of a smile or laughter.
Try to start every morning with a smile – it releases the happy hormones.**

Henry points to a red butterfly fixed to a tree, which tells me to go straight ahead. Then, like the others, he disappears as quickly as he came. Why do they all vanish so quickly? I stand there with the smile symbol in my hand and put it away in my rucksack with the other symbols and quotes I've collected. I put my hand in my pocket and am overjoyed to feel all ten marbles rolling around. I've gained two marbles through smiling and laughing!

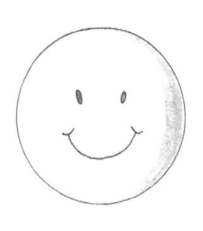

'Right, Angela,' I think to myself. 'Make a promise to include a bit of fun in your life. You deserve it after all you've been through.' I refocus my mind on reaching the Butterfly Mountain. Where my focus goes, my energy will flow. No more getting caught up in anyone's else's stuff! I have enough of my own, thank you very much. The vision of my golden bubble and blow-up sumo wrestling suit makes me smile. I must stay focused on my reward.

Key points

- Your body doesn't know the difference between what's real and what's not. It will respond in the same way whether you're running from a lion, watching TV or listening to something. It will put you into the fight or flight response.

- Breathing techniques help to put you into the rest and repair response. They calm and centre you and increase oxygen levels to reach every cell.

- Protect yourself with a bubble in whatever colour you wish. Visualise it surrounding you and letting other people's negative thoughts and energy bounce off you.

- If you're a natural helper, start putting yourself first instead of everyone else. The only person who can change this is you.

- Be aware of your environment. This includes what you watch, what you listen to and who you talk to. Listen to other people's success stories. You're in control of the next 24 hours, so use them wisely and be mindful of what you tell yourself.

- A smile can change your emotions. It releases the feel-good hormones such as endorphins and serotonin and calms the nervous system, putting you into the rest and repair response.

CHAPTER 3

CLARA CALM AND TOBY TIME

Pace yourself and define your day with moments of serenity

I walk past the red butterfly feeling even more focused on my mission to reach the Butterfly Mountain with all ten marbles in my pocket. Where my focus goes, my energy will flow. Lexi is trotting by my side with a spring in her step, tail wagging. The sky is now a brilliant blue and the sun is shining. It's such a change from a short while ago when it was all dark! I can feel the warmth of the sun's rays against my skin, loading me up with vitamin D and serotonin, the happy hormone. I smile and remember what I was told about smiling and how it can change your mood. There have certainly been days when I've lost my smile. I didn't think I had anything to smile about. I've been so wrapped up in my own illness that it has pushed everything else aside. But when I smile now, I feel more connected to myself, lighter and happier.

I love being in nature and find it therapeutic. As I walk, I notice my surroundings – the trees and the gnarled bark encasing them. I bet these trees have some stories to tell. They look ancient, with interwoven branches projecting like long, wrinkled fingers narrowing at the ends. I go to the nearest one and press my hands against it to feel the bark. I gently wrap my arms around it and hug it. It feels as if the tree is hugging me back. I've heard that hugging a tree is good for you because it releases a hormone that makes you feel calmer. I lay my head against the tree, close my eyes, breathe slowly and smell the bark. It's such a calm and relaxing feeling, almost spiritual. I'm not religious but it gives me a feeling of connection with nature. I push my ear against the bark and can almost hear the tree talking to me.

I gently come away from the tree and start rolling the magic marbles around in my pocket. They give me such a feeling of empowerment and remind me how to use my energy wisely. I carry on walking and think of the mission I've been given. It starts to feel a bit daunting. Feelings of doubt begin to creep into my mind again. What am I doing? Where am I? Will I ever reach the Butterfly Mountain? What if I arrive with less than ten marbles? Will I ever get better? Why do I keep doing this to myself – self-sabotage! I'm so good at it – I should get a medal for such an unhelpful and unproductive thought process but I can't seem to stop myself. It's exhausting. The negative thoughts keep whirring around in my head. I feel as if I'm playing a tennis match – yes, I can reach the Butterfly Mountain; no, I can't; yes, I will get better; no, I won't. My hand wraps around the marbles and I start counting: one, two, three, four, five, six, seven. I've lost three marbles just through my thoughts! I stop, put my head in my hands and feel emotion welling up inside me. I'm good at doubting myself, questioning what I've done and lacking self-belief. How can I quieten these thoughts and stop playing this constant tennis match?

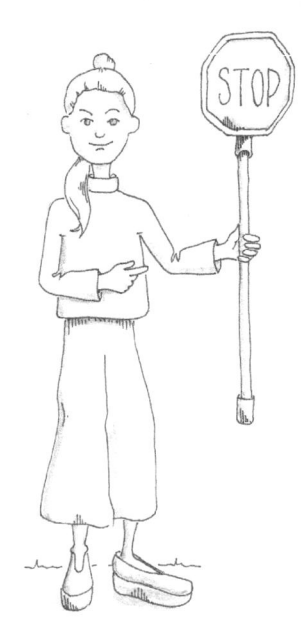

Just as I'm wondering

what to do, I notice a woman coming towards me. Her dark hair is in a ponytail. In her hand is a black cane with a STOP sign embedded in the top of it. Is this another person who's here to help and guide me? The woman introduces herself as Clara Calm, a psychologist. She asks if I'm having trouble with thoughts going backwards and forwards like a tennis match.

'How did you know?' I ask.

'Because you hold the magic marbles,' she says, 'and they're powerful.'

In a soft and gentle voice, she says, 'When negative thoughts come up and you feel a tennis match playing out in your head then just acknowledge those thoughts; be aware of what's happening in your mind. It's so important to recognise the thoughts and not to try and push them away. Thank them but let them know you don't need them anymore – don't let them have the power. Try the STOP technique. This is when you must firmly say stop by pushing your hands forward as if you're stopping someone coming towards you. Come into the present moment and think about your feet on the ground and take a few deep breaths. Feel your ribs rising and falling, your belly pushing out and sinking back in. Then observe your thoughts; don't judge them, just acknowledge them. Then proceed by changing your focus to a different thought. Another way is to notice the thought and then to tell it to go away.'

I think about my thought patterns as if my head is moving from left to right. I acknowledge them, thank them and then shout 'STOP' and push my hands out in front of me. I focus on my breathing, deep breaths in and out, and feel my feet connected to the ground. I change my thoughts and focus and say out loud, 'I *can* complete this mission, I *can* get better and I *will*.' I focus on my breathing – four breaths in and six out through pursed lips. I feel reconnected with the ground and a sense of calm and stillness fills my mind. I think again about my end goal –

to get the marbles to the Butterfly Mountain. I feel more positive and confident and suddenly all ten marbles are back in my hands again.

Clara smiles and gives me the STOP sign from the top of her cane. As she hands it over, she says this symbol is to remind me of the technique. She also gives me a card, which I look at straight away:

The STOP technique
S – Stop
T – Take a few deep breaths
O – Observe your thoughts – acknowledge them
P – Proceed – change your focus

She tells me I need to practise the technique, then points to a tree. There on the bark is another butterfly pointing the way – but this time in sky blue. I put the STOP sign into my rucksack with the other symbols and cards. I stop to take out the other symbols and remind myself of all the techniques I've been shown so far.

1. Butterfly from Hugo Hope, to remind me of being hopeful, keeping my focus and using my energy wisely.
2. Bellows from Barbara Bellows, who showed me breathing techniques.

3. Golden bubble from Billie Bubble, to protect myself from others and be aware of my environment; what and who I listen to, read, watch, talk to.
4. Smile from Henry Happy, reminding me that a smile can help release my happy hormones.
5. STOP sign from Clara Calm reminding me of the STOP technique.

They're great techniques and so easy to do. I can't help myself and start singing Meatloaf's 'Paradise by the Dashboard Light'. I love this song. I keep singing and it feels good. I haven't sung properly on my own for ages as I've not felt like it, but boy does it feel great. In fact, it feels brilliant! I know that singing is a great mood lifter and can stimulate something called the vagus nerve but I have no idea what that is or what it does. Anyway, it feels good so it doesn't matter.

What I'm being made aware of by all the people I've met so far is the power of the mind. Until now I didn't appreciate how powerful thoughts are and the impact they can have, not only on my mind but also my body and energy. It makes me realise that staying in my negative thought pattern is never going to help me to heal. Having a few ideas on how to move forward is so helpful. I gather my thoughts, call Lexi and follow the sky blue butterfly sign. 'OK, Angela,' I think to myself, 'stay focused and keep thinking of what you want.'

After all that singing I set off feeling good. It has certainly lifted my mood. I feel better as if I have more energy. I start skipping and hopping and notice a group of people behind me, chatting but also running together. They look as if they're really enjoying themselves. There must be about 20 of them. As they pass, one of them grabs my arm and pulls me along. I start running, and I'm loving it! I feel as if I'm blowing the cobwebs away. I've not run for such a long time. This is amazing. No sooner have I started than my usual competitive nature takes over and I'm pushing towards the front, wanting to be first. The front runner is going at quite a pace and I struggle to keep up. Lexi is running beside me and she's panting too. I'm now seriously out of breath and can't keep going. I must stop. I bend over to get my breath back and collapse onto a bench. The group carry on past me, running and chatting.

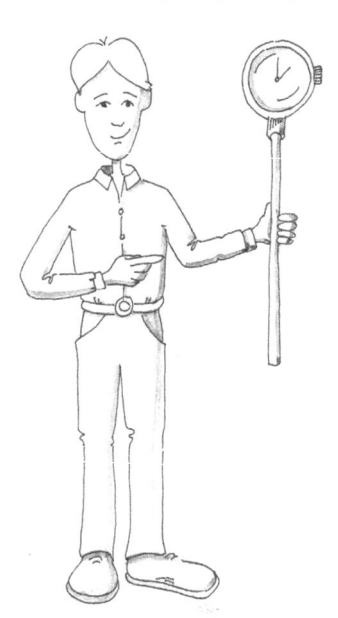

'Angela, what are you doing? What are you thinking? Why are you always so competitive – always pushing yourself?' I say to myself, with my head hanging down. I think one of the runners has stopped beside me but when I look up, I see a middle-aged gentleman wearing a stunning blue suit and holding a cane in his left hand. On the top of the cane is a watch. He sits down beside me and introduces himself as Toby Time. The first thing I notice is his piercing blue eyes, which remind me of Paul Hollywood's from *The Great British Bake Off*. He waits patiently while I get my breath back. Lexi is also still breathing heavily.

'How are you feeling?' he asks.

'Exhausted,' I admit. While I say this, I put my hand in my pocket and can only feel four marbles. I count again just to check. Yes, only four. 'Oh no,' I think to myself. 'What have I done now?'

'I know what your mission is,' says Toby. 'You need to get to the Butterfly Mountain. But will you have enough energy if you push yourself like this?'

'Good question,' I say. 'Probably not.'

'If you push yourself too hard, you'll crash,' he says, 'and you won't have enough energy to get to the Butterfly Mountain. You need to keep a steady pace that's manageable for you. I know that before you started this mission you said you were low on energy so if you want to achieve your goal, taking things easily and steadily is vital. Sticking to a baseline and pacing yourself is crucial for recovery. You want to avoid peaks and troughs of recovering for a short while, pushing then crashing and repeating the same cycle over and over again. I can't stress enough how important this is.'

He tells me to be mindful and to listen to my body, not my head.

'Your head will always try to talk you into things that you probably shouldn't be doing.'

'That's my problem, exactly that – pushing myself.'

'People who crash or get CFS are often overachievers. There is a personality type associated with this called the achiever pattern. These people push and drive themselves, putting their bodies under continual stress, which means they stay in the fight or flight response. They behave as if they have something to prove to themselves or others – but you don't have anything to prove. All you need to do is to be true to yourself.'

My breathing calms and I thank Toby for his wise words. Before he goes, he reminds me about the story of the hare and the tortoise. 'The hare charges off at breakneck speed and thinks he's so far ahead he'll just take a nap. Meanwhile the slow and steady tortoise takes his time. Having regained his energy, the hare wakes up and gets to the finish line just after the tortoise crosses it. Slow and steady wins the race. Charging ahead loses the race. In your case, this is not just the race to the Butterfly Mountain but also the race to your recovery.'

Toby gives me the watch that sits on the top of his cane to remind me of the importance of taking it slow and steady, finding my baseline and avoiding crashes. I put it in my rucksack with the other symbols and quotes. He points to the fence, where an orange butterfly is indicating the left fork in the path ahead. He wishes me luck, hands me a card and carries on along the path, whistling. When I turn around, he's vanished. I must remember that I'm in a magical world and never know what's going to happen next! I'd never have been able to run like I just did in the 'real' world. Maybe there is hope. I look at the card:

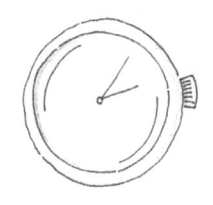

Remember to pace yourself and take it easy.
As the tortoise said to the hare –
SLOW AND STEADY WINS THE RACE.

I put my hand in my pocket and feel all ten marbles again. I love their texture and the way I feel when I connect with them. I feel drawn to them; I can feel their power and strength and this fills me with fresh determination. I close my hands around them and see the Butterfly Mountain and the lake but this time in all their amazing colours. It's as if the marbles have just painted the landscape. The flowers are in shades of pink, orange and yellow; the sun is bright yellow and the lake is a brilliant blue. I can't wait to get there. Where my focus goes, my energy will flow. I want to make sure that I use my energy wisely so I can reach this paradise. I stroke Lexi and follow the left-hand fork in the path.

Key points

- Walking in sunshine helps with the production of vitamin D and the happy hormone serotonin, which also helps with sleep.

- Being in nature lifts your mood, helps with stress and makes you feel more relaxed, which puts you into the rest and repair response. Hug a tree!

- Use the STOP technique when your negative thoughts are spinning round in your head: Stop, Take a few breaths, Observe your thoughts, Proceed.

- Singing and gargling are two ways of stimulating the vagus nerve, which helps to calm you down. The vagus nerve connects the brain to the gut.

- Find your baseline and stick to it. Pace yourself to avoid the crashes and conserve your energy. Use a weekly planner, which may help you to stick to your baseline.

- Personality types include the achiever pattern, which makes you push and drive to achieve and prove that you're capable.

CHAPTER 4

FELICITY FOOD

Think of food as your medicine

Being out in the sunshine lifts my mood. All my senses are alive – I can smell the trees, feel the ground beneath my feet and the gentle breeze on my face. I can hear the leaves rustling in the wind and almost taste the gorgeous fresh air. As I think about my sense of taste it makes me realise how thirsty and hungry I am. I've been walking for a while now and haven't had anything to drink or eat. I come across a flat, welcoming piece of grass and remember that I have a small blue and yellow blanket in my rucksack. It has been there for ages and I'd completely forgotten about it until now. It was given to me by Catherine when I first started struggling with my energy. I take out the blanket, lay it on the soft grass, sit cross legged and open my rucksack again. I rummage around and find a can of cola and a couple of chocolate biscuits.

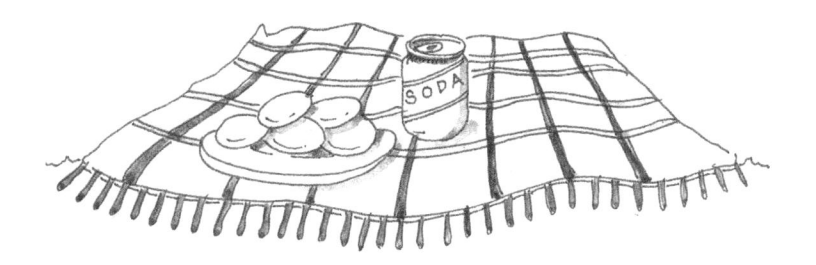

'Perfect,' I think to myself. 'This will help me to feel more energised so I can continue my mission.' I admire the view and enjoy the sunshine while eating and drinking. 'This feels good,' I think to myself as I let my face absorb the sun's rays and enjoy the warmth on my cheeks. I'm feeling so relaxed. I automatically put my hand in my pocket to check the marbles. I only have four! Why have I lost six marbles? Hugo Hope told me that I would gain marbles when I do things that will give me energy and lose marbles when I do things that will rob me of energy. Surely drinking the cola and eating the biscuits will be giving my body energy? I'm so confused.

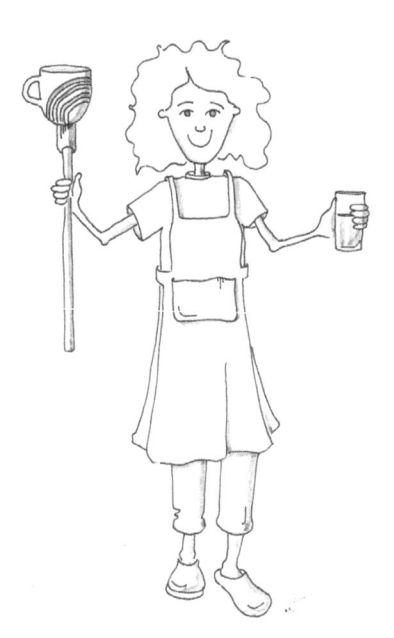

At that moment a cheerful young woman wearing a chef's apron appears from behind a hedge. She's holding a black cane topped by a cup that's decorated with a rainbow. She introduces herself as Felicity Food, a nutritionist.

'I know you've just lost six marbles,' she says. 'Do you know why?

'No,' I respond with a sigh.

'It's because of what you've just been eating and drinking. I'm going to help you to understand how food can put you into the fight or flight response or the rest and repair one. You've just put your body into the fight and flight state by drinking the cola and eating chocolate biscuits.'

'I thought cola would give me energy – a quick sugar fix,' I tell her.

She looks at me and says, 'I'm wondering whether you know roughly how many teaspoons of sugar there are in a can of cola?'

'About five?'

'I was shocked when I was first told,' she says, 'but there are more than 16! The body does need sugar to produce energy but not in such high doses and not in this processed form.'

'Wow, I had no idea! That's a hell of a lot of sugar – 16 teaspoons.'

'Sugar in this form is called refined sugar. It's inflammatory and acts as a stimulant, which puts the body into the fight or flight response. That's why you've lost the marbles! The same is true for such things as coffee, tea, alcohol and artificial sweeteners. So you may be having a nice chat with a friend over a cup of coffee and a sticky bun and thinking you're putting your body into a restful state but internally your body is putting itself into the fight or flight response. If you drink a lot of colas or have many teas and coffees, then switch to herbal teas, try decaffeinated or just reduce the number of cups you consume. Sugar also impacts your immune system, which needs to be functioning well because it helps to protect your body against infections. The best way to consume sugar is in its natural state in fruit, vegetables and grains such as oats. When you eat sugar in its natural state, it's absorbed more slowly into the bloodstream and is mixed up with fibre and nutrients. The sugar in a can of cola will be absorbed quickly into the bloodstream, causing a sharp increase in blood sugar that will initially give you a surge of energy but will be followed by a sugar crash, which can lead to physical symptoms such as fatigue, headaches and anxiety. So if you're craving sugar, it's better to eat a piece of fruit such as a kiwi fruit or an apple. Your chocolate biscuit will also be high in processed sugar and artificial sweeteners so will have the same negative impact on your body.'

'Gosh,' I say. 'I had no idea that food played such a key role in putting me into these responses. I've never thought about it like this before. I think of eating as something you must do rather than what it's doing to my body.'

'Your body is only as good as the food you put into it,' says Felicity. 'Think of food as your medicine. That will help you when it comes to making choices about the food you eat.

Follow me so I can show you more and help you to get some marbles back.'

I follow Felicity around a hedge. On the other side I can see two ornate chairs at a long wooden table. Felicity invites me to sit in the large, almost throne-like chair at the top of the table. When I take a closer look, I see that the table is completely covered in food – everything imaginable in all different shapes, colours and sizes. What a spectacular sight! I can't quite believe what I'm seeing but then I remind myself that I'm in a magical world.

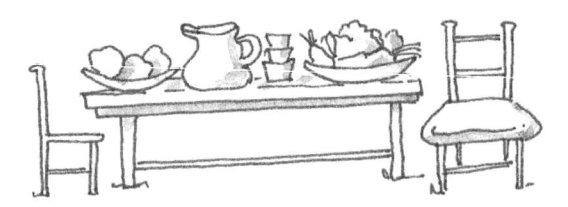

'Welcome to my banquet, Angela,' Felicity announces. 'I'm fully aware of your mission but you need to make sure you have enough energy to get to the Butterfly Mountain, which means eating and drinking the right sort of food. We eat to give us energy and help us grow and repair. Every cell in your body needs food – but it must be the type of food that will support you rather than create problems for you. The big question is, what is good food? I'm going to help you with this. Now, before we start, I think you should get yourself hydrated, so drink that beautiful pint of filtered water in front of you. I've given Lexi some too. Water will help to put your body into the rest and repair response because your body consists of 70 per cent water. It will help to nurture your amazing cells. Trying to do the basics well is so important when it comes to food, starting with water. It's the most basic of them all but it's vital and often forgotten.'

I pick up a pint glass that looks like a stained glass window and start drinking the water. I can feel my whole body thanking me for hydrating it.

'All of your 40 trillion cells will be thanking you,' says Felicity. 'Water is essential to life. If you're dehydrated, you're putting your cells under stress. It's also good to hydrate your digestive tract before you eat. This is a hollow tube that passes from your mouth all the way through your body. It's where digestion takes place. You can't digest properly if your body is in the fight or flight response. If you drink a pint half an hour before you eat it gives the body time to absorb the water, hydrating its cells and the digestive tract, ready for the food to be processed.'

She reaches down and picks up two toy alligators and a miniature football goal. It makes me giggle and wonder what on earth is going on. But then she continues. 'Your digestive tract is the length of two normal-sized alligators or a standard football goal – about 25 ft long. And that length of tract wants to be hydrated.'

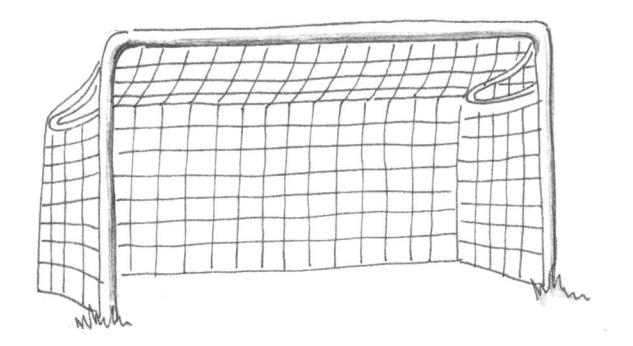

Ah, now I get it.

'While you're drinking your water, I'm going to tell you a story, so listen carefully. Imagine you're on an organised boat trip to a desert island. You arrive at the island, look around for a while and when you think it's time to leave you go back to the boat. But the boat has gone without you and there isn't another one for a month. You can't get off the island. There's no food or water. It's very hot and there's no shade. How would you feel?'

'Scared, petrified and frightened that I wouldn't survive.'

'Exactly, and that's how your body and cells will be feeling too. You're going to be in a panic wondering how on earth you're going to survive for a month until the next boat arrives. Out of nowhere a pint of water appears and you quickly gulp it down with a huge sense of relief and gratitude. But afterwards you'll start to worry. Will any more water turn up or is that it? A couple of hours later, another pint of water appears. You drink it with a great sense of appreciation. This continues. Every now and then a pint of water appears, ensuring that you're fully hydrated. How do you feel now?'

'I think I'd feel reassured that I'd have water and would survive.'

'That's exactly how your body and hence your cells feel when they have enough water – reassured. It reduces internal stress, restores health to your cells and their membranes and helps to improve the flow in and out of the cells. If you drink water regularly then your body won't feel like a desert island. Ideally you should drink a pint of water when you wake up and then regularly throughout the day but never more than one pint in any hour – and don't drink for half an hour before eating. If you drink immediately beforehand then all you do is flush the food down and through the tract without letting the nutrients get absorbed properly and your body doesn't hydrate properly. Aim for four pints a day, spread out, but take it slowly to start with. You can also eat food that's hydrating such as cucumbers, watermelon, soup, casseroles and smoothies.'

I mull this over for a while and realise I need to make sure that I keep myself hydrated. I put my hand in my pocket and feel that I now have six marbles – I've gained two just by drinking enough water. 'Wow that's amazing,' I think to myself. 'That's easy to do; I can manage that.'

'As you can see I have two signs at the end of the table, one that says "Rest and Repair" and the other that says "Fight or Flight",' continues Felicity. 'I'm going to give you an item of food and you need to decide which label it should go under. If you get it wrong, you'll lose a marble but if you get it right, you'll gain one. The purpose of this game is to help you understand which foods you need to focus on more. Here's a common breakfast cereal covered in pasteurised milk. Where are you going to put it?'

I take it from Felicity and put the bowl under the Rest and Repair sign but as I do this, I feel two marbles disappear from my pocket.

'I've just lost two marbles. I thought cereals were good for you?'

'You've just lost two marbles because some cereals are heavily processed and have had ingredients such as refined sugar, table salt, artificial flavourings and sweeteners added to them, which your body would prefer not to have. We've already talked about the impact that refined sugar can have on the body and it's the same for artificial flavourings, sweeteners and salt, which put the body back in the fight or flight response. Prevent blood spikes and create sugar balance by eating a variety of foods, including fats, carbohydrates and protein. If you eat a meal without protein, fibre or fat then your blood sugar will drop, leading to a sugar crash.'

She hands me a chart that lists all the different categories of food and the healthy options to look out for [you can find this in the resources section later].

'If you can, use rock salt or pink Himalayan crystal salt instead of table salt as that can be heavily processed too,' she continues. 'Some people struggle to digest cow's milk, so using plant milks such as almond or oat milk can be better for them.'

She hands me a bowl of porridge made with organic oats, cinnamon and plant milk and topped with blueberries and grated apple. I immediately put it under the Rest and Repair sign. As I do this, I feel two marbles materialise in my pocket!

'Porridge is great for you first thing in the morning. Or make it the night before by soaking the organic oats with plant milk and spices such as cinnamon. Put it in the fridge and eat it the next morning topped with fruit such as blueberries and grated apple, which contain many valuable nutrients. To make it even easier, top it with frozen fruit before you put it in the fridge overnight. Blueberries are full of what's called antioxidants, which are good for the body and can prevent illnesses.'

Felicity hands me a ham sandwich made with white bread, which I put under the Rest and Repair sign. But as I do so I feel two marbles disappear.

'White bread is a processed, refined food stripped of fibre and nutrients and may have additional ingredients such as sugar,' Felicity explains. 'White bread causes large blood sugar spikes, which I've already told you put your body into the fight or flight response. Again, be kind to yourself. If you can, eat wholemeal brown bread or sourdough, which contain more vitamins, minerals and fibre and don't give you such a sugar spike. Your body will respond the same way to other refined foods such as white pasta, white rice and white potatoes as it does for white bread. Try swapping to unrefined foods such as wholewheat pasta, brown rice and sweet potatoes. Maybe try some pasta made with chickpeas, lentils or peas, or some alternatives such as quinoa, buckwheat, red lentils or rice spaghetti.'

'Hmm,' I think to myself. 'I'm not sure but I'll give it a go.'

Felicity goes on to say that some people with CFS do better on a gluten-free diet but it's not for everyone. 'Gluten is found in some grains, including wheat, barley and rye. Keep a diary and see how you react to it. If it affects you, give it up for a couple of weeks and see what happens.'

She hands me a bowl that looks as if it has all the colours of the rainbow in it. It's a gorgeous colourful salad full of roasted vegetables. When I put this under the Rest and Repair sign marbles reappear in my pocket! I'm getting the hang of this.

Felicity asks, 'Have you heard of the expression "eat the rainbow"?'

'No.'

'It's good to eat as many different colours of fruit and vegetables as possible because each one provides a different health benefit. Maybe try a new one each week. The recommendation is to eat up to 30 different varieties a week but take it slow and steady. Don't eat 30 in one day if your body isn't used to it! I've put a few of my favourites on this plate – green leafy vegetables, carrots, different salad leaves as well as radishes.'

Felicity hands me a bottle of vegetable oil. I take it and put it under the Rest and Repair sign but feel some marbles disappear again. I'm confused again. I thought the body needed oil.

Felicity explains.

'Oils such as sunflower oil and vegetable oil are known as hydrogenated or trans fats. Heating them up makes them toxic and creates inflammation in the body so they should be avoided if possible because they'll put your body into the fight or flight response. The best oils to use are coconut oil or olive oil that's cold compressed and stored in a dark glass bottle. Try to avoid fried foods because they're usually cooked in vegetable oil at high temperatures.'

I ask Felicity if I've got the right idea. 'So you're telling me to eat lots of different fruit and vegetables as each one has a different health benefit – and to think of eating the rainbow. Try to eat foods in their natural state and avoid those with lots of things added to them. Reduce sugar and processed, refined foods such as white bread, pasta and rice and eat wholewheat or wholegrains. The body needs good fats, which can be found in foods such as avocado, almonds and chia seeds. Try to cook with olive or coconut oil.'

'You've got it,' says Felicity. 'Take it slow and steady. Try making a couple of changes when you can. But I want you to be kind to yourself and not beat yourself up all the time about what you should or shouldn't be eating. The best way to think about it is to remember the 80:20 rule. Eat well 80 per cent of the time and 20 per cent of the time eat what you like and enjoy it. But do it with knowledge. Put in the good stuff and gradually reduce the stuff that you think may not be helping you.'

Felicity puts a large bowl of soup in front of me. It's made with butternut squash, carrot, onion, sweet potato and red peppers and is topped with coriander. She also gives me a colourful salad to eat with a delicious home-made dressing. I sit down to eat and realise I'm starving.

'Eat slowly, chew every mouthful and savour every moment,' she says. 'When you're in the rest and repair response your body can digest properly. That includes the state of mind you're in when you eat as well as whether you're eating on the run or sitting down and eating in a relaxed way. You may find that eating smaller portions throughout the day may help, say every two to three hours.'

After eating all this delicious food, I put my hand in my pocket and feel for the marbles. All ten are there once again. Lexi also has a bowl of healthy dog food. Felicity sits down next to me and gives me her cane topper – the cup with the rainbow on the side – and a card that says:

Remember that food is your medicine.
Eat with knowledge and love.

'The cup is to remind you to drink water and the rainbow is to remind you to eat the rainbow. If you want to be the best you can possibly be, brimming with health and happiness, then it's what you put into your body that counts.'

She gives me a bottle of water to take on my journey. I put the rainbow cup into my rucksack with the other symbols and the card. Felicity points to a tree, upon which sits a beautiful purple butterfly pointing straight ahead. Off I go with Lexi on to the next stage of my journey to the Butterfly Mountain.

Key points

- Hydration is important. Try to drink up to four pints of filtered water a day – spread it out throughout the day, never drink more than one pint in any hour and don't drink for half an hour before eating. Your body consists of 70 per cent water. Take it slowly over time.

- Eat sugar in its natural state in fruit, vegetables and grains. Use pink Himalayan crystal or rock salt and olive or coconut oil. Eat healthy fats such as avocado, almonds, chia seeds, flaxseeds, pumpkin and walnuts.

- Avoid processed sugar and stimulants such as tea, coffee, artificial sweeteners and alcohol as they put your body into the fight or flight response. Avoid or reduce refined food (white bread, white pasta, white table sugar, processed foods, cakes, biscuits) as much as you can. To avoid sugar spikes, swap to unrefined foods such as brown rice, wholemeal pasta, buckwheat and quinoa.

- Eat the rainbow. Try to gradually increase your fruit and vegetables, maybe up to 30 different varieties, as they are full of key nutrients. Eat whole, natural foods.

- Eat slowly and mindfully and chew every bite so that the body can digest the food properly while you are in the rest and repair response.

- Remember the 80:20 rule. Eat well 80 per cent of the time.

CHAPTER 5

NATHAN NIGHT

*A good night's sleep helps
the body to heal*

After a healthy meal, I'm fully nourished and hydrated and ready to set off again. I'm so lucky to have such a loyal companion in Lexi. I keep my mind focused on the Butterfly Mountain. I wonder what the reward will be when I get there. I smile to myself, hoping it will be worth it. As I continue on my journey, clouds start forming, darkness begins to fall and I can feel the odd spot of rain against my cheek. The wind has also started to pick up and the dark clouds overhead begin to affect my mood. I feel more tired and less upbeat. Despite feeling a bit low, I'm determined to keep going. Out of the corner of my eye I see Lexi disappearing off down a right-hand fork in the path. She'll be back soon; she always is. But as I carry on, I notice she's no longer with me.

I call her name but she's nowhere to be seen. I call again – still no sign of her. I decide to turn back and follow the path that I last saw Lexi disappearing down. As I continue, the path becomes narrower, the trees get closer together and I start to feel claustrophobic. I keep calling for Lexi as I go deeper into the woods but there's still no response. I start to panic as I'm beginning to feel lost. I can no longer see the clouds above and the darkness seems to be encroaching on me. I can hear noises all around me – the snap of a twig, the rustle of the leaves. I can feel my mind going into overdrive wondering who or what is following me. My heart rate increases, as does my breathing, and I'm beginning to feel scared.

'Lexi,' I shout, almost screaming her name. I can feel the tears building up behind my eyes. Why am I here? What am I doing? Another noise, another twig breaking behind me. I turn round and feel my heart hammering in my chest. I stop and am about to scream when I see a deer running away. Where is Lexi? This is so unlike her. I'm now surrounded by trees that all look the same. How on earth am I going to get out of this? Am I ever going to find Lexi? Am I ever going to get to the Butterfly Mountain? I start to panic again as my heart rate and breathing rate increase. I put my clammy hand into my pocket and realise that I've lost five marbles. Here I am, back in the fight or flight response. I stop, take off my rucksack and reach into it. I pull out the first symbol I can find – it has the word STOP on it. My mind is in a fog and I'm struggling to think straight. Why do I have this sign? And then I remember the STOP technique. This might help me to get out of the spiral of negative thoughts. I remember to acknowledge my thoughts and not try to push them away but thank them. I shout 'STOP' to myself and push my hands out in front of me. I take some slow, deep breaths in and out, four breaths in and six breaths out, pulling in my belly as I breathe out. I think about my feet on the ground, being connected to the earth. I start to feel a bit calmer and then observe the thoughts that are coming up as well as my emotions – the fear of losing Lexi and being lost in the woods, of never reaching the Butterfly Mountain, of never recovering from CFS, of never having a life again… it just keeps snowballing on and on. I shout STOP again, take another deep breath, reconnect with the ground under my feet and try to change my thoughts. 'I will find Lexi and get out of the woods. I will get to the Butterfly Mountain. I am going to recover from CFS.'

I can still feel my mind reeling so I shout out loud, 'Just eff off!' I repeat it three times and that feels much better. In fact, I can feel a small smile starting in the corners of my mouth. The smile grows and soon my whole face is filled with this smile. I feel calmer, more focused and more positive. I notice that my heart rate and breathing rate have come down. I put my hand back in my pocket and notice I have all ten marbles again. I feel so proud of myself! The power of the mind is amazing.

I've never really paid much attention to all this before but I now realise what you say to yourself can have huge consequences. I put the STOP symbol back in my rucksack and think about Lexi. I focus on finding her. I call her name again but this time calmly. I start to walk back the way I think I've come, although I'm not sure. Then I hear a bark and there's Lexi at the bottom of a tree, barking at the squirrel that's halfway up it. Thank God! What a relief. I call her and she comes trotting over without a care in the world. I stroke her lovingly with sheer relief. Lexi looks at me wondering what all the fuss is about. I've found Lexi; now I need to focus on getting out of the woods. It's totally dark now and I'm struggling to see in front of me. I'm not going to think about how I'm going to do it but just believe I will. I take a deep breath and follow my intuition. After a short while I notice that I'm no longer in a dense wood; the trees are getting further apart and I can see a clearing. I continue walking and soon I'm out of the woods and back on a path. I breathe a sigh of relief.

I'm proud of myself again – it feels good to be achieving things, regardless of how small. What I'm realising is that focusing on the smaller things that need your immediate attention can help, especially if the bigger picture seems too overwhelming. As I walk along the path, I recognise my surroundings. It feels like déjà vu until I realise that I'm back where I started, looking at the purple butterfly on the tree. How frustrating! This feels like the story of my life – going round in circles and getting nowhere fast. I slump down at the bottom of the tree and realise how tired I am. I've really pushed myself today. I don't think I have the energy to carry on. It's been a long day. I open my rucksack and find another can of cola. I know that Felicity Food advised me against sugary drinks but right now I don't care. I'm so tired and need a fix. I know I shouldn't but I do it anyway. Then I start wondering where I'm going to sleep...

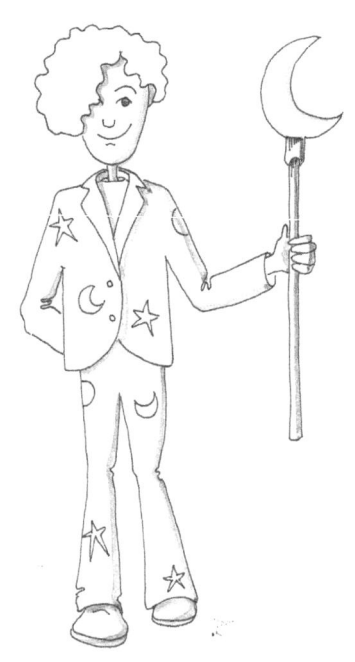

I'm sitting with my head in my hands when I feel a tap on my shoulder. The tap comes from the end of a cane that's attached to a young man. He is holding a black cane with a silver moon on top. He introduces himself as Nathan Night, a sleep expert. He asks me if I'm looking for somewhere to stay.

'How do you know?' I ask him.

'Because you have the magic marbles,' he says. 'Follow me. You can sleep in my cottage.' He helps me up and lends me his cane so I can use it as a crutch.

He has an amazing inner light that seems to project outwards and makes shadows fall across our path. I follow him, with Lexi by my side. We go back into the woods as I lean on his cane to help me to walk. Then I see his cottage, which looks similar to mine. It looks so inviting. It has a thatched roof and lights all around it, with a path winding up to the front door. Smoke is spiralling out of the chimney and the door is magnificent with a big, crescent-shaped moon embossed on it. Nathan pushes the door open and it looks so cosy and warm inside. As we enter, I can see a gorgeous, welcoming fire. I sit down next to it in an old rocking chair. The fire is hypnotic, with the flames dancing in front of my eyes. Lexi curls up at my feet, enjoying the warmth. Nathan sits by the fire opposite me in a beautiful chair that's covered in some of the constellations. He hands me a pint of water to drink. Mustn't forget to keep hydrated! It may undo some of the harm I've done by drinking the can of cola. I'm now cross with myself for drinking it, knowing the impact it will have on my body. I slip my hand into my pocket to discover that I've lost six marbles!

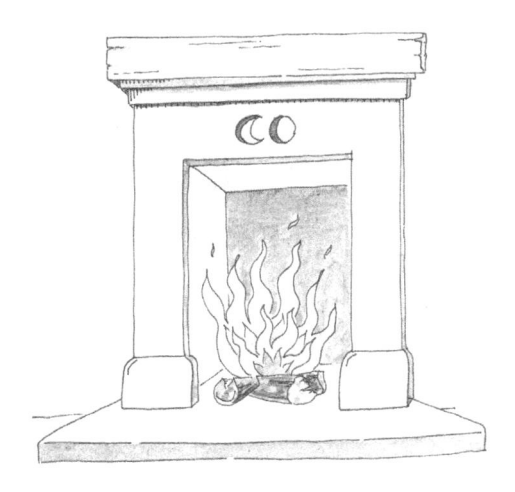

Nathan starts telling me how crucial sleep is to recovery. He says it's the chance your body gets to rest and repair and asks me how I've been sleeping.

'I'll be honest and admit I've been struggling. Even though I feel so tired I just can't seem to get to sleep. It's so frustrating. And if I do get some sleep, I still wake up completely shattered and it's a fatigue that's so difficult to describe.'

'I'll give you a few tips that may help,' he says. 'There are a few things you can try. Establish a routine – go to bed at the same time and get up at the same time each day. Stop using electronic devices an hour before going to bed – blue light from these devices suppresses the hormone melatonin, which is known as the sleep hormone. Listen to relaxing music, do a meditation or have a warm bath with magnesium salts. Many people with CFS have the same problem – they either struggle to get to sleep or have unrefreshing sleep and wake up exhausted. Sometimes that's because their bodies are still in the fight or flight response. The most important thing is to try to put your body into the rest and repair response before you go to bed as well as during the day, so try not to consume stimulating drinks after noon.'

'Whoops,' I think to myself. 'Drinking that can of cola won't have helped.'

'Sometimes sleep meditations can help,' continues Nathan. 'Doing activities throughout the day that will put you into the rest and repair response will impact your sleep – maybe not straight away but with time, when your body is less wired. Would you like me to do one with you now?'

'Yes please! That would be lovely.'

I move onto the sofa and he puts a blanket over me that's covered in moons and stars. He advises me to close my eyes and just listen. He has a slow, hypnotic voice that's very relaxing. He then delivers a beautiful, relaxing sleep meditation. His calming tones are so soothing. I can feel my whole body relax and let go. All I can do is focus on the words he's saying and my breathing. I can't remember the last time I felt this relaxed and sleepy.

I put my hand in my pocket and can feel all ten marbles

again. I just hold them and feel their smooth surfaces. They help to keep me focused on the end goal of reaching the Butterfly Mountain and finding my reward. Then he shows me to a sweet little spare room with an inviting bed. I lie down and close my eyes and can feel myself drifting off to sleep.

I sleep in fits and starts – I'm annoyed with myself again about the cola but do some deep breathing exercises to keep me relaxed and stop myself from getting anxious. I also tell myself to forget about it and move on. Overall, it's a slightly better night's sleep but I'd love to be able to have a full night's sleep and wake up feeling refreshed. I'm sure with time it will come – that's what Nathan has told me. Next morning, at the bottom of the bed I can see the moon symbol from Nathan's cane with a card that says:

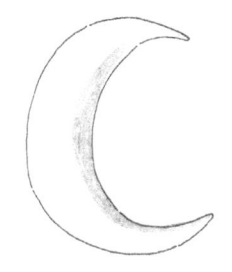

Never give up – sleep will come.
Just believe it will and be kind to yourself.
As you recover, so will your sleep.
Just remember to keep yourself in that rest and repair response.

Despite Nathan's kind note my mood is still low this morning. I feel frustrated and despite everything I'm still cross with myself for drinking the can of cola. Also, chasing Lexi and going off the path means that I've gone round in circles. I'm not sure I'll ever get to the Butterfly Mountain. I feel exhausted and fed up and just want to stay in bed. So I do.

Key points

- A good night's sleep can help aid recovery. If you must have caffeinated drinks, then try not to have them after lunch.

- Put your body into the rest and repair state before sleep and also during the day.

- Go to bed at the same time each night and get up the same time each morning.

- Stop using electronic devices at least 60 minutes before sleep. Blue light suppresses the melatonin production needed for sleep.

- Doing a meditation or a breathing technique can help before going to bed as this will put you into a relaxed rest and repair state.

- Have a warm bath in the evening with 500 g of magnesium salt and stay in it for 15 to 20 minutes.

CHAPTER 6

HANA HABIT AND MILO MOVEMENT

Healthy habits and movement to connect the mind and body

I'm struggling today. My mind is in a bad place and I feel shattered. I know I did too much yesterday by chasing after Lexi and getting myself all wound up and then stupidly drinking that can of cola. Having CFS is so frustrating. I just feel like eating cake, drinking coffee and curling up, even though I know it will put my body into the fight or flight response. I can't think straight and feel exhausted. Maybe I'll just stay here in Nathan Night's spare bed. I think I'll just curl up and hide from the world. I can feel the tears welling up and I can't help but start crying.

I should be trying to get to the Butterfly Mountain but right now I don't have the energy and can't be bothered. The tears keep falling and I feel sorry for myself. I pull the blanket over my head and sob. My thoughts go round and round – why me, it's not fair, I'll never get to the Butterfly Mountain, I'll never find my reward... Then I put my hand in my pocket. I only have one marble! I'm running on empty – I've pushed myself, made stupid choices and because of this I've lost virtually all my magic marbles, all my energy. Mr Hope told me that I need all ten marbles to reach the Butterfly Mountain.

I feel a nudge. I pull down the covers and there's Lexi. She jumps on the bed and starts trying to lick me. I think she's checking in on me – she usually does. Then I notice that there are two people behind Lexi – Nathan Night but also someone I haven't seen before. She's holding a black cane and on the top of it is a tiny tree. She has a warm, gentle face. She comes over to me and gives me a huge hug. I can't help but melt into her arms. We stay there for a while as my tears continue to flow. It feels good just to have that human connection – to let someone in to hold and hug you, to be vulnerable and acknowledge that you're not coping and it all feels too much. After what seems like ages, my tears stop and we both sit up and look at each other. She introduces herself as Hana Habit, another therapist.

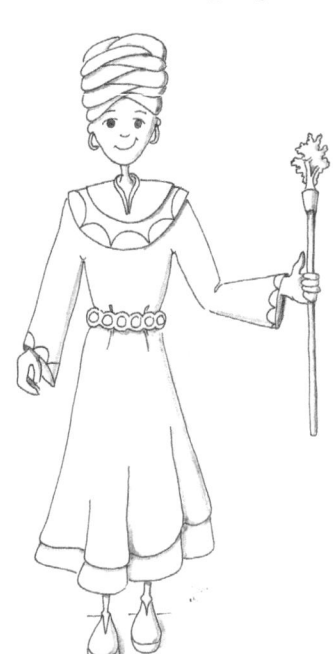

'It's OK to show that you're struggling,' she says. 'Being vulnerable is being strong and true to yourself. When you feel like this, let people in; let them know you need help and support. But most of all be gentle and love yourself. It's OK to have a bad day. Now let's focus on helping you to form helpful habits so that even when you're having a bad day these habits become automatic. They'll help your mindset, make you feel less wired and help you feel connected with yourself. Think of it like a tree. We're putting down roots to help the tree to grow. Trees need a strong foundation. They need light, water and food. If they don't have those things, they won't grow. The only person who can help you grow and change is you. You must take control of what you want. You must wake up every day fully committed to your recovery. You need to be living and breathing that thought every second of every day. You need to believe you can recover and reach the Butterfly Mountain.'

I get out of bed, sit by the fire and mull over what she's said. Nathan brings over a pint of water, which I quickly finish. He reminds me that all of my 40 trillion cells need to be hydrated.

'Let's start by thinking about how you can get out into nature every day, even if it's just walking around your garden or sitting outside,' says Hana. 'Then you need to focus on gratitude. When you're grateful for the things or people around you it has a huge impact. When you're being grateful, your brain won't let you have negative thoughts. Practising gratitude can have incredible effects on your immune system and mental health by helping you feel happier. It can also help with sleep. There are a few methods you can apply but for now just think of three things you're grateful for. This can be anything at all – people you're grateful for, good things around you, your community, nature. It can be as simple or as complex as you like. When you're thinking of them, I want you to truly appreciate them and recognise why you're grateful for them. Feel the gratitude with your whole heart, body and mind.'

I close my eyes and start to think. It's not easy if you've never done it before. My mind keeps going walkabout and I keep pulling it back into focus.

'The first thing I feel grateful for is Lexi. She's my faithful companion who's always by my side and looking out for me. And she never answers back! The second thing I'm grateful for is nature, especially the trees. They help to give me life. It felt wonderful when I hugged a tree. I'm grateful for the joy they bring through their changing leaves and the shade they give from strong sunshine. I appreciate their different shapes and sizes and their beauty. My third gratitude is for being in this magical place, having the opportunity to hear ideas that will help me. I'm sincerely grateful for all of this and I'm saying and feeling that with my whole heart.'

I automatically put my hands on my heart and feel the love and connection. I haven't felt like this for a long time. Hana then suggests that I write down the three things I'm grateful for. She hands me a sheet of brightly coloured paper and a rather beautiful pen that has 'Gratitude' written on the side. I write my gratitudes on the pieces of paper and Hana gives me a little jar with 'Gratitude' embossed on the side. She tells me to fold up the pieces of paper I've written on and put them in the jar.

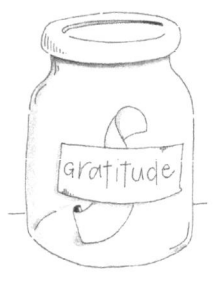

My three gratitudes
1. My dog, Lexi
2. Nature, especially the trees
3. Being in this magical place so that I can learn how to help myself.

'Great start,' she says, giving me another hug. She also says that I could write my gratitudes in a journal or just say them to myself as well as putting them in a jar, which I can then open and read when I feel the need.

'Loving yourself is powerful and helps you with self-worth,' she says. 'Truly loving yourself with your whole heart is so valuable and helps you to really connect with yourself. It shows that you value yourself. Now I want you to go over to the mirror on the wall and give yourself a high five.'

I walk to this beautiful mirror, which looks like a

full moon. Hana tells me not to say anything but just to look at my true self. I look at myself then slowly lift my hand to the mirror and give myself a high five. I feel very self-conscious as I do it.

Hana then turns to me and says, 'Why don't you do it again but this time with more conviction? Say to yourself, "I see you and I love you."'

I repeat the exercise and this time I smile and look at myself properly for the first time in ages. I notice my nose, mouth, my lank hair and my tired eyes. But this time I say to myself,

'I see you and I love you.' Saying 'I love you' to myself feels so hard. I'm not sure I've ever truly loved myself. I've loved other people and given them my love but I don't think I've ever said it to myself. I say it again with more conviction: 'I see you and I love you.' I high five myself again and this time I feel a warm surge throughout my body. I look in the mirror and instead of a drawn face I'm looking at a softer, warmer face with a bit of a glow. And do you know what? It feels good. I feel good. I turn round and see Hana smiling. She gives me a card and tells me it's a reminder to high five myself in the mirror every morning:

High five yourself every morning.
Start your day with a boost of positivity and momentum.
Stop seeking approval from others and give it to yourself instead. Love yourself.

I put the card into my rucksack and promise to do this every morning along with my gratitudes. While I have the rucksack open I peer inside to look at the other symbols I've collected – including the butterfly from Mr Hope. Seeing the butterfly reminds me of the Butterfly Mountain. Having done my gratitudes and high five I feel more positive and connected with myself. I'm going to make it to that Butterfly

Mountain. I see the bellows. I close my eyes and think of the breathing techniques I was shown by Barbara Bellows. I put my hand on my belly and breathe into my belly for a count of four then breathe out through pursed lips for a count of six. I repeat this a few times. It's such an easy technique but so effective in getting me into the rest and repair state. I see the golden ball and it makes me think of my environment and who and what I'm talking to. I feel grateful to Hana Habit, who's helping me to form morning habits and put my body into the rest and repair state. Nathan Night has given me the information about sleep. I'm in the perfect environment right now. The smile symbol catches my eye and I feel a smile spread across my face. A smile really does lift my mood. I feel another warm glow spreading through my body. I love it.

The STOP sign has already come in handy when I was lost in the woods and the watch is a reminder to pace myself. The cup with the rainbow on it reminds me of the importance of food, especially 'eating the rainbow', keeping myself hydrated and reducing processed sugar. 'Ah,' I think to myself, 'that needs a bit of work.' But this time, instead of beating myself up, I just smile.

Hana says, 'Expressing gratitude and performing a high five every morning are good habits to get into. They're simple, take little time but will have a huge impact on you. Another one is saying affirmations to yourself. These are positive statements that can help you to challenge and overcome self-sabotaging and negative thoughts. If you repeat them daily, you can make positive changes. So I want you to start with the question, "What if I'm good enough to…?" I want you to finish the statement. Come up with your own suggestion of what it is you want. My advice is to start with something simple and then you can make them more challenging. You can have more than one affirmation. Saying them out loud can help to reinforce the belief so repeat them three times.'

That's hard. What do I really want? What do I want to tell myself? I sit for a few minutes while I mull it over. I come up with a few ideas and start saying out loud, 'What if I'm good enough to really love myself with my whole heart and tell myself that I'm truly awesome and will get better.' Then I put my hands on my heart and feel connected to myself, even though I'm struggling to fully believe what I'm saying. I repeat this statement three times and each time I feel stronger and can hear my voice get louder the more conviction I have.

Then Hana says, 'At the beginning you may find these words hard to hear and they may not fully resonate with you now but the more you repeat them, the more you will start to believe the words you're saying. By loving yourself you're also loving all 40 trillion cells in your body.'

She asks if I have another statement and I almost shout, 'What if I reach the Butterfly Mountain and find my reward?' As I repeat this three times, I close my eyes and visualise the Butterfly Mountain and the lake. I can see them, I can feel them and in that moment I know that I will get there. Where my focus goes, my energy flows. My focus is fully on the Butterfly Mountain.

Hana then hands me another card on which to write my affirmations. This time she gives me a pen that has 'Affirmations' embossed on the side. I write down my affirmations and put them in my rucksack along with the pen. I feel so much better having carried out those three simple activities. Here are my two affirmations, starting with the words, 'What if I'm good enough to…':

… love myself with my whole heart. I am awesome and I will get better.
… reach the Butterfly Mountain and find my reward.

Nathan then produces a bowl of what looks like cold porridge. He explains that it contains oats soaked overnight and mixed with almond butter, almond milk, chia seeds, blueberries and raspberries. He tells me to make sure I eat it slowly and chew every mouthful until it liquidises in my mouth. He says that eating with love and gratitude impacts how your food is digested as it puts you into the rest and repair state.

Hana then gives me the tree that's on the top of her cane, along with a huge hug. Just before she goes she says, 'You must be committed to your recovery, to what you truly want. Only you can make that commitment to yourself.' With that she gives me a card and then walks out of the front door. This is what's written on the card:

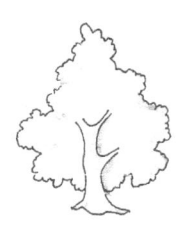

Habits change your mindset and your health and are the key to your future.

I'm about to pull my eyes away when I notice another person coming through the door. He's young, dressed in a tracksuit and holding a black cane. On the top of the cane is a small figure in a yoga pose. He introduces himself as Milo Movement, a physiotherapist and yoga teacher. He walks in, looks at me sitting slouched in the rocking chair and comes straight over to me. He smiles and starts to speak in a positive, energetic voice.

'OK, Angela, let's start at the beginning with your seated posture. I can see you're slouched down into this rocking chair. What impact do you think sitting like this is going to have on you, your movement and your body?'

I immediately sit up and he laughs, which makes me laugh too. It's hard to sit upright in a rocking chair, though! He suggests I change seats into a more upright chair.

'I suppose sitting in a slouched position could give me a sore neck and back but can it also impact my mood?'

'Absolutely,' says Milo. 'It will affect everything you've

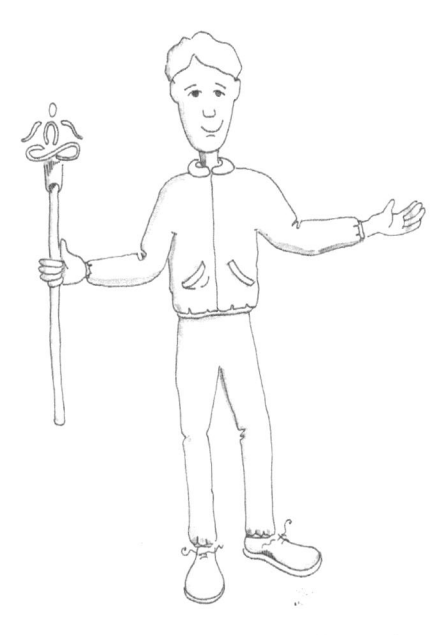

just mentioned. Good posture is vital to your overall health. It helps with your muscles, joints, breathing, nerves and blood vessels. I know you've been shown some breathing exercises that you can do lying down or sitting up but if you're slouching then this will influence how much air you can get into your lungs. Good posture helps to keep everything aligned so your body can move freely. Sitting up straight means having both feet on the floor with your shoulders relaxed and hips and knees at 90 degrees. Try to have your head over your shoulders. Your head weighs about 5 kg, so you want it to be supported properly by the structures around it. It's the same when you lie down or walk – you need good posture.'

I follow his instructions and feel the difference when I'm sitting up straight. He suggests I try the breathing technique – breathing in for four and out for six while sitting in a slouched position and then sitting upright – to compare how it feels. I notice the huge difference in how much air I can get into my lungs when I sit upright. He says that breathing exercises can really help as part of my morning routine, either lying down or sitting up and, if necessary, supported with a pillow in my lower back when I'm sitting upright. I continue to do my breathing exercises for the next ten minutes, with my eyes closed but sitting upright and supported in the chair and my feet connect to the ground.

Milo sits patiently while I continue breathing in and out. When I've finished, he talks about the power of the mind and body and how they can all come together with movement, but specifically with yoga. He says, 'Movement is needed for your whole body, however small or big you make the movements. Yoga is amazing – it helps with the connection between the mind and body as well as sleep, switching off negative thought patterns and much more. It also helps to put you into the rest and repair response. Have you done much yoga before?'

'A little – but not much.'

'Do you feel like doing some now?'

'I'd love to.'

He puts two yoga mats on the floor. We both sit cross legged on the mats and he reminds me to sit up as tall as I can. He starts with connecting with the breath, one hand on the stomach and the other on the heart while we breathe slowly in and out with our eyes closed. This is such a simple practice but feels so calming and it makes me feel at one with myself. He has such a soothing voice I can't help but let every word he says flow through every part of me. As I continue breathing, he talks about how yoga is meditative and can help every physiological process in the body. We then do some basic yoga moves flowing from one posture to the next in a slow, controlled and relaxed manner. Gorgeous is the only word I can think of to describe it. At the end of the session, he puts some blankets over me and conducts a ten-minute meditation with his hypnotic voice. I feel so relaxed.

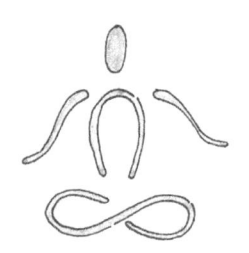

As he finishes the meditation, I lie there for a few minutes in a trance-like state feeling calm, relaxed and at peace. As I come round, I can feel myself smile as I feel such gratitude for all the practices I've been shown this morning. I sit up slowly and Milo comes over, sits beside me and gives me the figure in the yoga pose from the top of his cane. He says, 'This is to remind you of the importance of movement and posture. Movement such as yoga can be helpful first thing in the morning. It can keep you calm, help with mental focus and concentration, and the breathing exercise fills you up with fresh oxygen. Yoga and movement can help you get the lymphatic system moving first thing in the morning and can help your bowels.'

Then he hands me a card. Written on it are the words:

Yoga is not about touching your toes – it's about what you learn on the way down.

I start to put all the objects I've been given this morning into my rucksack. As I do so, I remind myself of the lessons I've learned by making a note of the symbols:

1. The tree symbol, reminding me of good daily habits
2. The moon symbol, reminding me of the importance of sleep
3. The yoga pose, reminding me of good posture, yoga and meditation.

Milo asks, 'How are you feeling now? I know that before you carried out these morning routines you felt at rock bottom because you'd lost nine marbles. You felt as if you'd crashed and were wired.'

'I know that this will all take time but right now I feel reconnected with myself,' I tell him. 'I feel calmer, more positive and more energised. I feel more focused on what it is I want, which is to get to the Butterfly Mountain and find the reward.'

I put my hand into my pocket and feel that all ten marbles have returned. I take them out, roll them around in my hands and observe the rainbow colours. My eyes are drawn to them and I feel their positive energy. I realise that I've put myself into rest and repair by doing all these activities with Hana and Milo. I'm so proud of myself! He places his hands over the marbles, wishes me luck on my journey, then disappears. Lexi licks my hand and Nathan Night and I walk out of the front door together. He walks me back to the purple butterfly, gives me a hug and I set off again on my journey to the Butterfly Mountain.

Key points

- Be kind to yourself, even when you know you've contributed to a dip in energy.
- Let others help you – showing vulnerability shows how strong you are.
- Love yourself with your whole heart.
- Get into good daily habits, including gratitudes, affirmations, high fives in the mirror, breathing exercises and meditation.
- Good posture in all positions helps the whole body.
- Yoga is good for mindfulness, getting into the rest and repair response and giving you a feeling of calm and connectedness.

CHAPTER 7

HARPREET HEALTH

A healthy gut rules the day

I set off feeling relaxed and calm with Lexi by my side. I feel better for having done all these activities – gratitude, yoga, meditation, high fiving myself in the mirror, to name a few. I feel lighter, more positive and more energised – much more energised. I'm now laser focused on reaching the Butterfly Mountain. In my mind I can feel and visualise this place, the peacefulness and spectacular scenery. I close my eyes just for a second to bring it to the forefront of my mind. I continue walking and after a short while I see another butterfly but this time in pink, pointing to the left.

It's a beautiful day and the path is clear. I can feel the sunshine on my face, giving me all that fabulous vitamin D. Being surrounded by nature feels so good and makes me happy. The path meanders through the trees and I can see the shadows they cast falling on the path and creating different shapes. The wood is full of stunning flowers, which remind me of the flowers around the Butterfly Mountain's lake. I put my hand in my pocket to feel the marbles. I'm convinced that these magic marbles have given me a boost of energy today.

The path then comes into a clearing and I can see a river. The water is bubbling over the stones and pebbles. As I walk further into the clearing, I can see a little girl running along, chasing butterflies. She looks about five or six years old and seems to be having a wonderful time, as if she doesn't have a care in the world. It makes me think of my own childhood – young and carefree, in that lovely 'innocent' state. There's also a woman sitting on a rug, watching the girl. A sense of freedom and fun just grabs hold of me as I throw off my rucksack and copy her by running around chasing butterflies.

Soon both of us are doing it together, running and laughing. In this state I can do anything! I can see a rope swing attached to a tree that's hanging over the river and can't help myself. I remember going on one when I was a child. I jump on and start swinging away. I'm having such fun and it feels brilliant. I can hear myself screaming with sheer enjoyment. I'm so engrossed that I fail to hear the woman shouting at me. Suddenly I hear a loud snap and the branch holding the rope breaks. It all seems to happen in slow motion. I hold on tight as the rope swing and I create a massive splash as we collapse into the river. The girl and the woman are both standing on the bank, laughing. Lexi is looking at me as if to say, 'What are you doing?' Once I surface and realise I'm fine, I start laughing too. I'm thoroughly soaked but don't care. I pull myself out of the river and lie on the bank. It feels good to laugh. I haven't had a good belly laugh for ages because I haven't had anything to laugh about. But now my sides are aching from laughter!

Once the hysteria has died down, the woman asks if I'd like to come over to their house and dry off. I jump at the chance. But just as I scoop up my rucksack, an apple and some grapes fall out. I put my hand in my pocket and feel two marbles disappear. The woman turns round and looks at me and it's only now that I notice that she's wearing a colourful shirt covered in all sorts of fruit and vegetables.

'I know you've just lost two marbles,' she says.

'But why have I lost two marbles? I don't understand.'

'Follow me up to the house and once you are dry, I'll explain it to you.'

She introduces herself as Harpreet Health, a gut health expert. She tells me her daughter's name is Joy. 'That's appropriate,' I think to myself. Harpreet looks as if she's in her mid-thirties, with straight black hair and a beautiful nose piercing.

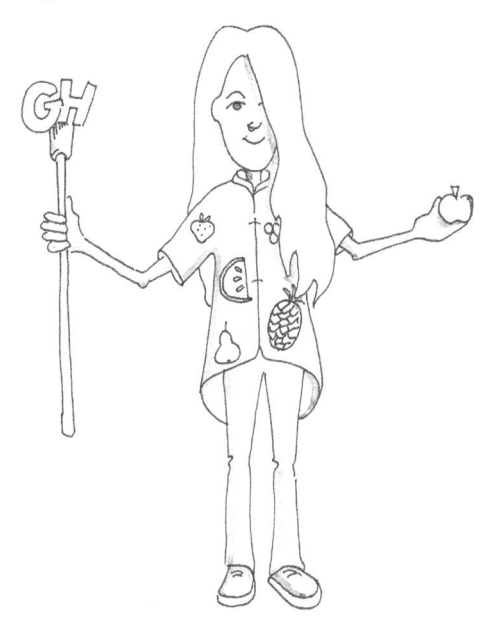

When we reach the house, I notice a black cane in the front porch – and on the top of the cane are the letters 'GH', which she tells me stand for 'Gut Health'. She grabs it as we pass by. As I look out of a window towards the back of the house, I see an amazing vegetable patch with all sorts of colourful plants growing in it. It reminds me of 'eating the rainbow'.

Harpreet tells me that she grows all her own organic

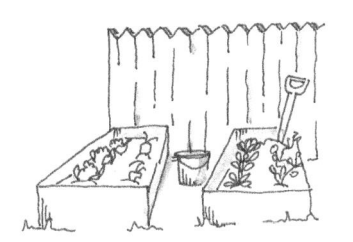

fruit and vegetables because she's trying to keep her body and gut as healthy and free from toxins as possible. She asks me if the grapes and the apple are organic.

'No,' I reply.

'Well, that's why you lost two marbles.'

'So what exactly does buying organic mean?'

'It means that the farmers don't use any pesticide – but if they do it's under strict guidelines, with no artificial fertilisers and healthier soil. Organic, locally sourced, seasonal fruit and vegetables are the best. Let me tell you about the Dirty Dozen and the Clean 15. The Dirty Dozen are fruit and vegetables covered with the highest level of pesticide residue and the Clean 15 have the lowest. So when you shop, if possible try to make sure that the Dirty Dozen are organic. The Clean 15 don't need to be organic as they don't tend to have as much pesticide residue on them. The reason you lost two marbles is that apples and grapes are part of the Dirty Dozen and have the highest levels of pesticide residue.'

'Can't you just wash it off with water?'

'You can wash some of it off but not if it gets into the flesh of the plant or into the root system. But that's a good point. You should always wash fruit and vegetables before you eat them.'

Harpreet leads me over to the vegetable patch and says, 'I'd like you to choose five different fruit and vegetables you think belong in the Dirty Dozen category and five that you think belong in the Clean 15 category. If you get it right, you'll gain a marble but if you get it wrong, you'll lose one.'

So off I go to collect my ten fruit and vegetables, five for each category. Harpreet has put two bowls on the table, one marked 'Dirty Dozen', the other 'Clean 15'. I place the fruit and vegetables into the two bowls. When I take out the marbles, I see that I've lost a further two. Harpreet explains that I put avocado and asparagus in the Dirty Dozen bowl when they should be in the Clean 15 bowl and spinach and peppers in the Clean 15 bowl when they should be in the Dirty Dozen bowl. I move them to the correct bowls, feel my pocket and find that all ten marbles are back again. Harpreet hands me a chart as a reminder [you can find this in the resources section].

'But,' says Harpreet, 'please don't worry if you can't buy organic. It's still better to eat non-organic fruit and vegetables rather than none. Now let's talk about my favourite topic, gut health. A healthy gut is crucial and will help you with your recovery. As Hippocrates said 2,500 years ago, "All diseases begin in the gut."'

'What exactly is the gut and what does it do?'

'You must have heard various expressions about the gut such as "You have guts", meaning you're brave; or "Spill your guts", meaning reveal everything. Or you have gut feelings, emotions that feel like the intuitive truth. This is because the gut is connected to the brain via the vagus nerve. The gut is your digestive system, which was discussed earlier by Felicity Food. The gut is important because it helps your body to function. But most people think of the gut as the intestines. If one adult's intestines were laid out, the small intestine would be around 6 metres long and the large intestine about 1.5 metres. The gut's main functions are to digest food, absorb the ingested nutrients and then excrete the waste. The key point here is that you're only as healthy as the foods that you put into your body. For example, proteins are the building blocks of life; they help to repair and build your body's cells. The gut helps in so many ways, for example with energy production, hormone balance, skin health, mental health, elimination of waste and toxic substances, disease protection and more. Seventy per cent of the immune system lives in the gut and that's why gut health is so important to recovery. Also, the gut provides about 95 per cent of the body's serotonin, the happy hormone. Remember that you're only as healthy as your gut.'

'But how do you know if you have a healthy or unhealthy gut?'

'Another good question,' Harpreet replies. 'If it's healthy then you'll have good bowel movements, good energy, normal gas and little bloating, good clarity of mind and healthy reactions to food and stress. If your gut is unhealthy then you may experience digestive issues such as excess gas and bloating, irritable bowel syndrome, sleep issues, fatigue, skin problems, poor concentration, moodiness and other conditions.'

'So what can I do to improve my gut health?'

'I love your questions! But this time I want you to do the work and to come up with some of the answers.'

Harpreet grabs two jars. One is labelled 'Healthy Gut' and the other is labelled 'Unhealthy Gut'.

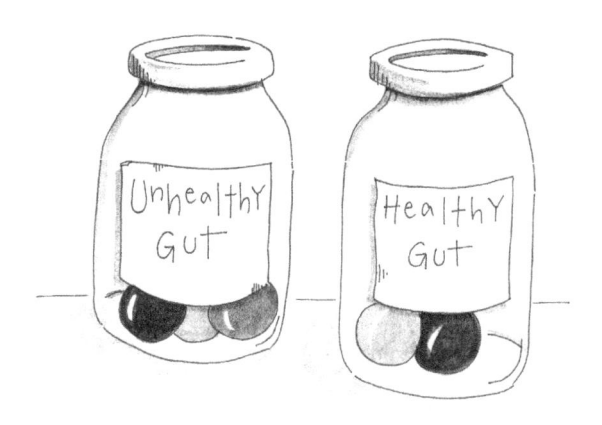

'Now I want you to use your magic marbles to find the answers. They'll play your journey so far like a movie, so you can pull out the key information you need. When a marble shows you something you think is relevant to gut health, put it into the relevant jar. Don't worry if you run out of marbles, as I have more here. The key thing to remember is what Hugo Hope talked to you about – the rest and repair response or the fight or flight one. Which do you think the gut needs to be healthy?'

'The rest and repair response,' I reply.

'Exactly!'

I start gazing at the marbles. I pick one up and start watching myself right at the beginning of my journey, getting stressed and anxious when I didn't know if I could complete this mission.

'Would this marble go into the Unhealthy Gut jar?'

'Definitely. Stress has a huge impact on your gut. It puts your body into the fight or flight response.'

I drop the marble into the Unhealthy Gut jar and as I do so the word 'Stress' appears on the surface of the marble. I pick up another one. This time I watch Barbara Bellows helping me with breathing techniques.

'Does this marble go into the Healthy Gut jar?'

'Absolutely.'

I drop this marble into the Healthy Gut jar and as I do so I see the word 'Breathing' appear on its surface. This is a genius way of helping me to understand what helps my gut. I continue like this, watching the replays of my journey and putting the marbles into the two jars. As I continue, I realise that gut health is related to your mind and body – your thoughts as well as what you eat and drink.

I start thinking about food and drink. I smile as I see myself drinking that can of cola and the number of teaspoons of sugar in that can – 16! That will certainly go into the Unhealthy Gut jar. As I drop the marble in, the word 'Sugar' appears on the marble.

'A diet high in processed foods and sugar can decrease the number of good bacteria in your gut,' says Harpreet. 'This can lead to chronic inflammation throughout the body, resulting in several illnesses, so it has a massive impact on your gut health. Your gut loves fruit and vegetables so eat the rainbow, as Felicity Food told you. They are high in fibre and your gut loves fibre.'

When I've finished, I stand back and look at the marbles in both jars and Harpreet hands me a chart as a reminder:

Healthy gut (rest and repair)	Unhealthy gut (fight or flight)
Breathing	Stress and anxiety
Pacing and keeping to your baseline	Pushing and driving – achiever pattern
Hydration	Dehydrated
Unprocessed natural foods	Sugar and processed foods
Fruit and vegetables and fibre	Limited fruit and vegetables and fibre
Eating slowly, mindfully and chewing	Eating quickly or on the run
Oils – olive oil and coconut oil	Trans fats – vegetable oil and fried foods
Wholemeal foods (unrefined)	White bread and pasta (refined)
Sleep	Lack of sleep
Habits such as gratitude and mindfulness	Negative thought patterns
Yoga, good posture, meditation	Poor posture, lack of movement

'I hope this helps you to understand how you can support your gut. Now, let's talk about the microbiome. Have you heard of this?'

'A little but I don't know much about it.'

'The term gut microbiome refers to the microorganisms living in the gut. Each person has about 200 different species of bacteria, viruses and fungi living in their digestive tract. It's important to maintain a balance of good and bad bacteria. Too many bad bacteria and too few good bacteria creates an imbalance that's called dysbiosis, which can lead to ill health. It means you have too many of the pro-inflammatory species and too few of the good ones, which you definitely don't want! Dysbiosis can cause many issues but fatigue is a key one. You can't extract the goodness from food without good gut function. One way of looking after your gut is to supply it with foods that will feed these good bacteria. They feed off a sort of fertiliser called prebiotics, which are in many fruit and vegetables including bananas, asparagus, Jerusalem artichokes, onions, leeks and garlic. To increase the number of these friendly bacteria, eat fermented foods that contain live bacteria and yeast, known as probiotics. Examples of probiotic foods are kimchi, sauerkraut, miso and tempeh. But again, try these new foods gradually because you don't want to irritate and overwhelm the gut if it's already struggling. You don't need much to make a difference.'

Harpreet hands me another chart to take away:

Prebiotic foods (fertiliser)	Probiotic foods (fermented foods)
Bananas	Kimchi
Asparagus and leeks	Sauerkraut
Jerusalem artichokes	Miso
Onions and garlic	Tempeh

'Eating these foods may also help to rebuild the gut lining, which has often been damaged. If it has, it can create something called leaky gut, which means that unprocessed food particles and toxins can pass through the gut lining into the body, causing inflammation that will put your body into the fight or flight response. But it also means that you can lose healthy bacteria that line the gut and help with the absorption of nutrients from partially digested foods. You can repair this lining by eating the correct foods and cutting out the inflammatory ones.'

Harpreet asks me to follow her outside. She picks up a hosepipe and says, 'Think of your digestive tract like a hosepipe. When I turn on the water you can see that it all stays in the hosepipe and passes all the way through the hollow tube.'

She then picks up a second hosepipe and turns it on. I can see that there must be holes in it because water is spurting out of the sides.

'This hosepipe is leaking water through small holes just like it would with someone who has a leaky gut. So looking after your gut lining is as important as your gut health.'

All this talk of gut health makes me realise that I need the bathroom. I notice I'm a bit constipated. My bowel movements are a little uncomfortable to pass and take time to come out. When I finish, I put my hand in my pocket and realise I only have six marbles. How does being constipated take your energy? This doesn't make sense.

Harpreet looks at me and asks if I'm OK. I tell her about my constipation and the marbles disappearing. She explains that having a good daily bowel movement is important to my health and my gut because it stops the build-up of toxins, which put the body under stress and into the fight or flight response. Well, I must admit, I wasn't expecting to be thinking about my bowel movements when I started out on this journey!

'When you're constipated, toxins remain in the body for longer and can be reabsorbed back into the body, which you don't want,' explains Harpreet. 'It's important to have a good bowel movement every day. You know you've had a good bowel movement when you've passed your stools easily and feel as if you've had a full evacuation. People don't talk about it enough but it's so important.'

I ask her how to make sure I have good bowel movement and she tells me hydration is a great place to start. Then I realise I haven't had any water since I left Nathan Night's house. I've only had one pint today and I should have had four. Harpreet hands me a pint of filtered water and I feel all the marbles returning.

'Eating chia seeds soaked in water for ten minutes with a slice of lemon and a little pink Himalayan crystal salt is good for you, as well as plants that are high in magnesium such as spinach, peas, fruit such as avocados, bananas and blackberries, and wholegrains such as oats and brown rice. The more plants you can eat in their natural state, the better it is for your gut health, immune system and bowels. I'm going to make you something you can take with you to eat on the way to the Butterfly Mountain. Legumes are jam packed with fibre, so let's put in some of those. They're among the healthiest foods on the planet and they're cheap. But don't include them all in one go or they could upset your digestive system. They can become fermented and cause wind when the carbs are converted to methane gas. It's a good idea to soak the dried legumes in filtered water overnight before you cook them as they have tough skins that make the nutrients in them less accessible.'

'What is a legume?'

'A legume grows in a pod. Some popular legumes include black beans, chickpeas, green peas, black-eyed peas and kidney beans. Chickpeas are great and lentils have the thinnest shell of the legumes so are easier to cook and digest. They're also high in protein, fibre and nutrients, including iron.'

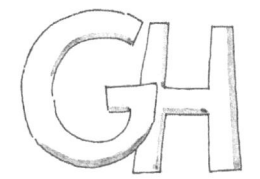

Harpreet disappears into the kitchen and returns with a colourful salad. I can see some roasted vegetables (red peppers, broccoli, tomatoes, courgette, aubergine), chickpeas, tempeh, lettuce, watercress, spinach, quinoa and sauerkraut. Harpreet says she has topped it with a delicious dressing of apple cider vinegar and extra virgin olive oil. She hands me the salad in a container that I put into my rucksack. Then she fetches her cane, takes the 'GH' sign off the top and hands it to me.

'This is to remind you of the importance of your gut health and bowel movements.' She also gives me a card that says:

As Hippocrates said 2,500 years ago,
'All diseases begin in the gut.'
Looking after your gut is looking after you.
Treat it kindly.

Harpreet takes me back to the path and shows me a brown butterfly. I smile and give her a hug before heading in the right direction.

Key points

- Gut health is crucial to recovery. The gut digests and absorbs nutrients that come from the foods you eat. The gut contains 70–80 per cent of the immune system and 90 per cent of your serotonin, the happy hormone.

- The microbiome is made up of microorganisms in the gut that include good and bad bacteria. Too much bad bacteria leads to dysbiosis, poor gut health and illness. Avoid inflammatory foods.

- Prebiotic foods act as fertiliser, feeding the good bacteria in the microbiome. Probiotic foods are fermented foods that build up healthy bacteria in the gut.

- Think of the Clean 15 and Dirty Dozen when deciding which organic fruit and vegetables to buy. Choose whole, natural foods and eat the rainbow to get the fibre the gut needs.

- For a healthy gut you need to put your body into the rest and repair response. Breathing techniques, yoga, meditation and good posture will all help.

- Have a good bowel movement every day and avoid constipation.

CHAPTER 8

HERBIE HOLISTIC

Understanding, nurturing and working with your body

My mind is buzzing but I keep reminding myself of where my focus needs to be – on the Butterfly Mountain. As I walk, I start to practise gratitude and try to stay in the present moment by feeling the ground under my feet and focusing on my breathing. Lexi is trotting along beside me happily enjoying all the different smells. I notice that the trees are thinning out and I can see further into the distance. The sun is shining and I feel good, especially because of everything I've learned about my gut. I have this vision of the microbiome looking like an army in my large intestine, recruiting the good guys into their regiment and marching on the fibre, breaking it down to release the nutrients to feed the good bacteria. The good bacteria then produce nutrients, which feed the cells in the colon and help to reduce inflammation. How great is that! All I need to do is feed my body with the food it needs to keep it healthy and not give it food that will stress it out and destroy the army of workers trying to look after me.

The trees are few and far between and I can see that the path is taking me downhill. In the distance I can see a village with an impressive church steeple. I wonder where the Butterfly Mountain is? I have to remind myself of Hugo

Hope's words – it doesn't matter how I get there; I just need to keep focused on my end goal. I feel good so I start running down the path with Lexi trotting by my side. I'm singing as I run and keep going until I'm on the outskirts of the village. I'm now out of breath. Hmm, maybe that wasn't such a good idea.

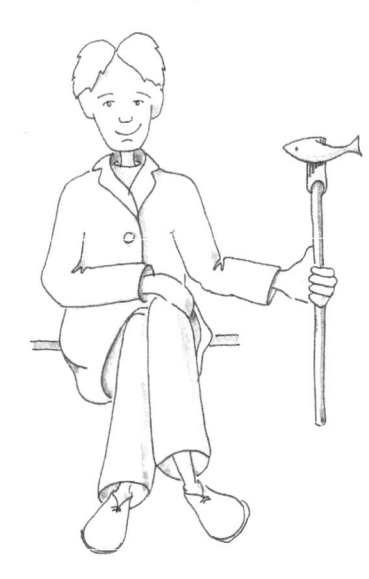

I continue to follow the path into the village and eventually it takes me onto a village green, where I can see two ponds side by side. I stop and look around. Sitting on a bench nearby is an elderly gentleman wearing a green overcoat and holding a cane topped with a silver fish. He turns to look at me with a warm smile. He waves his hand, beckoning to me to come and sit beside him. He introduces himself as Herbert Holistic – Herbie for short. I put my hand in my pocket and notice that I've lost two marbles. What have I done now? As I smile Herbie starts smiling with me.

'I know how it goes now. I must have done something to lose two marbles and I'm sure you're going to tell me how.'

'Yes, I will, but first I want you to look at both fishponds and tell me what you see,' says Herbie.

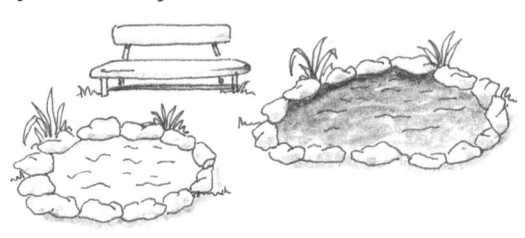

'One of the ponds is green with a lot of slime and you can see that some of the fish are struggling to swim,' I reply. 'The other is perfectly clear. You can see all the way to the bottom and there are fish swimming around in it freely.'

'Exactly. These two ponds represent you. If you put rubbish into your body with your thoughts and the food that you eat, it will look like the slimy pond. But if you eat well, become aware of your thoughts and look after yourself in mind and body, then inside you will look like the clear pond. I want you to think of the fish as being the cells in your body, all 40 trillion of them. The water that the fish are swimming in represents the fluid environment in which your cells live. Cells are so important! They're the building blocks of all living things. They form the structure of the body, take in nutrients from food that you eat and convert those into energy. They carry out numerous functions to keep you alive. That's why throughout your journey you've been reminded about how many cells you have and to look after them. You need to love your cells through your mind and body. You want your cells to be in the rest and repair response and not in the fight or flight state. Allow your cells to recover by giving them what they need. A cell membrane surrounds the cell, which protects it. Inside the cell are structures of different shapes and sizes that carry out different functions. These structures are called organelles.'

He pauses to allow me to take all of this new information in.

'Cells are amazing,' he continues. 'They're working all the time and know just what to do. They're all interconnected like a bustling community, just like the fish in the clear pond. There are processes going on in our body every second of every minute of every day that we pay no attention to. All these processes need energy. Think of a cell as a factory with several workers inside, each having a specific task to perform to make a product. If one of the factory workers is unable to perform their task then they won't be able to make the product effectively and efficiently.

In you, that product is a fully functioning, healthy cell. The factory workers in the cell are known as the mitochondria, which are powerhouses that produce the energy you need to live and breathe. They help you heal and strengthen your immune system and are like the batteries of each cell. The energy that powers every cell and organ in your body is produced by your mitochondria. When they don't produce enough energy then every cell is compromised and you'll feel fatigued. So it's very important to support your mitochondria. Consuming healthy food and drink is one way that you can really help them. Do you remember being told to eat the rainbow?'

'Yes,' I reply, 'Felicity Food and Harpreet Health told me about eating the rainbow.'

'Well,' he continues, 'all those colourful fruit and vegetables will support your mitochondria. Eating foods that are high in protein such as eggs, well-sourced fish and meat, nuts, seeds, lentils, beans and healthy fats will also help. You can support your mitochondria with exercise such as yoga and relaxation techniques that reduce stress, such as meditation. Keep to a baseline so that you're using your energy wisely while it's building up again.'

He hands me a chart to remind me how to support my mitochondria:

How to support your mitochondria	Description
Eat the rainbow	Colourful fruit and vegetables
Eat foods high in protein	Eggs, well sourced fish and meat, nuts, seeds, lentils and beans
Healthy fats	Avocados, coconut oil
Using your energy wisely	Stick to your baseline
Relaxing activities	Yoga, meditation

He asks, 'So do you know why you might have lost a couple of marbles?'

'I presume it's to do with energy. Is it because I ran down the hill using up precious energy that I need to get to the Butterfly Mountain? I remember talking to Toby Time about pacing and making wise choices about when and how to use my energy.'

Herbie lifts his stick and shouts, 'Exactly! Now let's go back to the ponds. Remember that the fish are your cells and the pond is the environment in which your cells live. Your cells are surrounded by fluid such as blood and lymph. If you think of the stagnant pond, how will the fish survive in this? What's creating that stagnant water?'

'Is it algae?'

'Absolutely. Algae thrive due to an imbalance of nutrients in the pond. They will eat off the sludge on the bottom of the pond created by fish waste, dead algae, leaves and grass. The imbalance can also be impacted by nutrients and toxins flowing into the pond from the surrounding soil. Algae can harm the fish too. So what do you think is going to create a poor environment for your cells? What's going to create that green stagnant water in your body?'

'I presume it's what I put into my body, including what I eat and drink. I learned a great deal from Felicity Food and Harpreet Health about eating and drinking food that creates a poor environment, such as sugar, highly processed foods, refined foods such as white bread and pasta, coffee, alcohol, trans fats such as vegetable oil, plus being dehydrated.'

'Yes, that's right. But your cells can also be influenced by your emotions, stress and negative, unhelpful thoughts. Gratitude and meditation can help with this. Your environment is also important. External factors such as cleaning or skin care products and soap can create toxicity, so choose these products wisely. Now, one day you notice that one of the fish in the green pond looks poorly so you take it out, give it some good food and then put it back into the same stagnant water. Is that fish going to improve and recover?'

'No. Because the unhealthy environment it was taken out of hasn't changed.'

'You're really getting it now!' says Herbie, doing a little jig. 'You can't cure the fish if you don't change its environment. If you don't change the water and get rid of the algae, and the food it's feeding itself, it won't recover. You need to take the fish out, empty the pond, clean out of all the sludge, protect the sides of the pond so that no external nutrients can affect its balance, fill it up with clean, oxygenated water, put some plants in the water and then put the fish back in. Only then will the fish survive. This is clearly demonstrated in the pond that is clear with fish swimming around in it moving easily. These fish are healthy. It's the same for your body and cells. You need to look at the whole environment. You need to look at all of yourself – what's influencing the body and the mind? Everything you've been learning along the way will help you understand how you can change your environment. If you don't do that you may struggle to fully recover. Like your factory, the workers all need to be working together to create the final product, which is you! But make sure you make these changes slowly and mindfully. Challenge your beliefs – but not all at once.'

'OK, I'm getting the picture. This journey has been amazing. I've learned so much and feel very grateful.'

Herbie goes on to tell me more about cells. 'The amazing cell membrane allows materials to pass in and out of it through small pores. It's selective, which means that not all substances can pass in and out. The health of the membrane is crucial. Substances such as carbon dioxide and toxins that are the natural by-products of metabolic processes going on in the cell pass across this selective membrane. It's important to get these toxins out of the cell and out of the body. You've already discovered how to get rid of toxins through daily bowel movements, deep breathing and keeping the lymphatic system moving. Sweating through exercise or saunas can help, too. Toxins can also be removed through urination. If the cell membrane gets damaged, the cell could potentially die. Eating a healthy diet will impact the health of the cell membrane. It particularly loves food rich in essential fatty acids such as oily fish, olive oil, seeds and nuts – especially walnuts, leafy green vegetables, flaxseeds, chia seeds and water. The fish need healthy food, just like your cells.

'Your liver also needs support. It's another organ that's so critical to recovery. All your blood is filtered through the liver – more than a litre every minute. The liver is responsible for receiving and processing all nutrients that enter the body. If you have energy issues such as CFS, which weakens your immune system, the liver's ability to filter nutrients properly will be affected and this will make your symptoms worse. The liver is our detoxifying organ; it helps to remove toxins from the body. If you overwhelm the liver, toxins can get reabsorbed back into the body, which you don't want. So my question to you, Angela, is how do you think you can impact the functioning of the liver? What do you think may stress the liver and make it work harder than it needs to, which will use up or waste precious energy?'

'Hmmm. Let me think. I presume it's the same as for everything else, whether it's your gut health, your cells or your mitochondria.'

'Yes. Go on.'

'Things like sugar, white flour, trans fats, caffeine, alcohol and processed foods.'

'You're spot on. Those will all put your liver into the fight or flight response because it's having to work so hard. Smoking also puts a huge strain on your liver, as does stress. So what do you think will help your liver?'

'Fresh fruit and vegetables that are as organic as

possible, to reduce the residue from pesticides that Harpreet Health told me about. Also probably nuts, seeds and keeping hydrated. But also doing things to help with stress such as walking outside in nature, exercises, breathing techniques, yoga, meditation and gratitude.'

'Absolutely. Foods high in omega-3 help to boost the liver's ability to filter waste. The liver loves berries and cruciferous vegetables such as cabbage, brussels sprouts, cauliflower and kale as well as beans, wholegrains and garlic. Green tea is full of antioxidants, which are helpful for liver health. Filtered water with fresh lemon squeezed into it can also help. It's important to stay hydrated to help flush toxins out of the body.'

Herbie hands me another helpful chart:

How to support your liver	
Organic fruit and vegetables Remember the Dirty Dozen and the Clean 15	Specifically berries, cabbage, cauliflower, kale, brussels sprouts, garlic
Foods high in omega 3 (essential fatty acids)	Oily fish, chia seeds, leafy green vegetables, flaxseeds
Nuts and seeds	Especially walnuts
Hydration	Filtered water with fresh lemon, green tea
Reduce stress	Nature walks, yoga, meditation, gratitudes, smiling, hugging a tree, breathing techniques

'The message is coming through loud and clear,' I say with a big smile.

Herbie holds his cane up high and shouts out, 'Eureka! I think she's got it!'

I remember the salad I was given by Harpreet, which

I have in my rucksack. I'm starving now! I take out the container and offer some to Herbie, who graciously declines, telling me he's already eaten. This is the type of food that will support my cells, mitochondria and liver. I eat slowly and mindfully, chewing every mouthful while thinking of three things to be grateful for, which puts my mind in a positive state. I think of the goodness the food is bringing into every cell of my body. When I finish, I put my hand in my pocket and can feel all ten marbles again. Yippee!

'I want you to listen very carefully,' says Herbie. 'I don't want you to worry and feel overwhelmed about changing things all at once. Do it gradually. Start putting in the good stuff slowly and you'll begin to see changes but they'll take time, so be patient. Think of a cup full of water. Drop some dirty soil into it and swirl it around so the water changes colour. How are you going to get the dirt out of the cup now?'

'Pick it out with a spoon?'

'You'd think so, wouldn't you? But the best way is to just keep filling the cup with clear water. As you continue to pour water into the cup, the dirt eventually pours out over the top of the cup and in time you're left with a cup full of clean water.'

'That makes so much sense to me,' I tell him. 'Just keep filling my body with the good stuff and over time it will help to get rid of the rubbish.'

Herbie asks how my journey is going and I tell him I have no idea where I'm going or how I'm going to get there but I know that I will. He then gives me the silver fish off the top of his cane and a card, which reads:

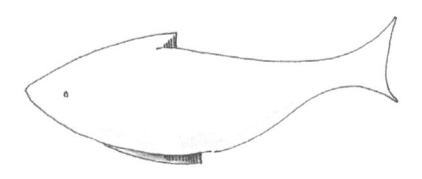

**The quality of your life is dependent on the quality of the life of your cells.
Learn to love your cells and therefore love yourself.**

He suggests that Lexi and I follow him, so we do. He takes us past the ponds, through a gate and into a wood. He points to a white butterfly on a tree. When I turn round, he has gone.

Key points

- Cells are microscopic and carry out numerous functions that keep you alive.

- Inside the cells are small organs called organelles, including the powerhouse known as the mitochondria, which produce energy.

- What you eat and drink can influence your mitochondria as well as wellness practices such as yoga and meditation.

- Your cell membrane loves essential fatty acids such as oily fish, nuts and seeds like chia seeds.

- Look after your lovely liver as one of its functions is detoxification.

- Look after the whole of you, body and mind, to thrive and survive.

CHAPTER 9

THE BUTTERFLY MOUNTAIN

Lexi and I follow the path in the direction indicated by the white butterfly, which takes us down into a valley. I enjoy taking in the scenery, the smells and the sounds. The shape of the valley begins to change and the hills on either side of me are getting taller, reaching up to the sky as if they're trying to communicate with each other. The sun is shining, which is creating shadows everywhere. This is a truly beautiful walk that gives me a chance to continue with my positive thoughts, my gratitude and just being in the present moment.

A clearing appears in front of me. I walk towards it and begin to see an expanse of water. It reveals itself to be a lake. When I reach the water's edge I become aware of butterflies flying around me. There's also a reflection in the lake – the silhouette of a mountain, which takes my breath away. I realise that I've arrived at my destination. It's exactly as Mr Hope described – the Butterfly Mountain and the lake, with so many beautifully coloured butterflies filling the air.

I feel jubilant. I'm finally here! I can't quite believe I've made it. I feel excited and proud of myself for not giving up, for persevering when times were tough. I didn't think I'd ever get here but what a huge achievement. There were times when I truly doubted myself but I kept hearing Mr Hope's words in my head: 'Focus on the Butterfly Mountain and don't worry about how to get there.' It's only now that

I notice all the flowers surrounding the lake, looking like a colourful carpet. I just stand and stare.

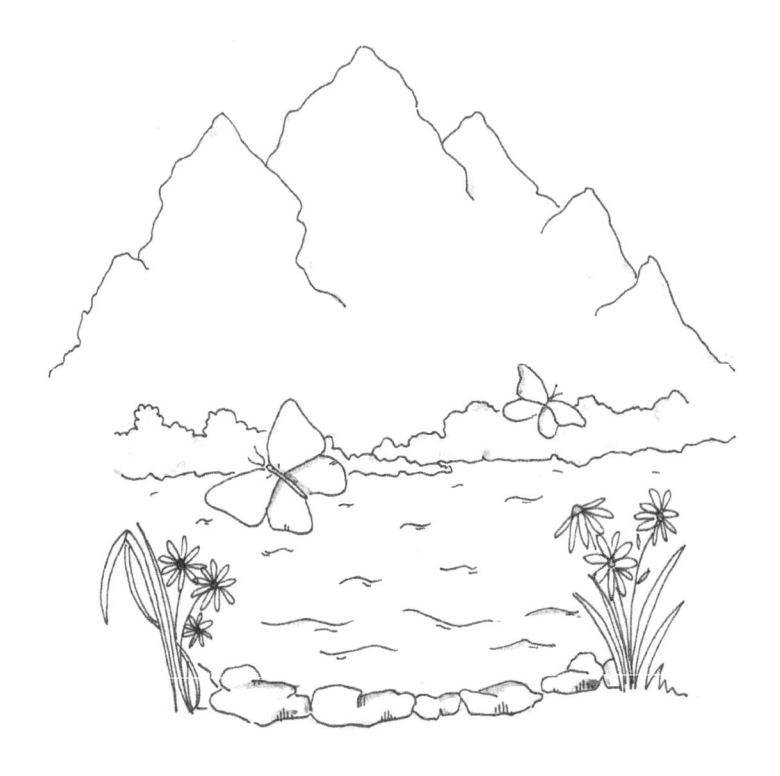

As I look ahead, I see the Butterfly Mountain, standing proud. As I take in my surroundings, I reach for the magic marbles in my pocket but they slide out of my hand. They begin to form a rainbow, starting at my feet and arching across the whole lake. As I look at this glorious vision it reminds me of a bridge. But a bridge has a definite end point and a rainbow doesn't. I'm still on my healing journey and the end is uncertain but I know I will get there. At the end of every rainbow is a treasure chest full of gold. Mine isn't full of gold – it's full of the techniques and things I can do to help myself that I've learned along this journey. I feel as if I have won a chest full of gold, though. I already feel more empowered and in control than I have for a long time.

I sit down on a grassy mound, take off my rucksack and empty out the contents. I lay out all the symbols I've collected along the way in front of me. I lift them up one by one: I start with the butterfly and roll it around in my fingers to remind myself of what it represents. Suddenly, I become aware of a shadow in front of me. When I look up, I see Hugo Hope, smiling. I stand up and he gives me a huge hug,

He says, 'You made it. I knew you would. The butterfly I gave you was a symbol of hope, of never giving up, and it helped you to focus on what you want. This whole journey was about looking at ways you can help yourself to get out of the fight or flight response and into the rest and repair one so that your body and mind can heal.'

I'm curious about the reward he mentioned when we first met.

'Ah yes,' he says.

He takes my hand and we go down to the lake. We kneel next to it and start looking into the water. At first, I see very little but the more I keep my eyes fixed on it, a picture starts to form. I can't quite believe what I'm seeing – it's me but I look so different. My hair is bouncy and glossy, I look happy and I have a broad smile on my face. My eyes are sparkling and I look radiant. What an extraordinary transformation.

'This is your reward – the ability to see the changes you've made,' says Hugo. 'You're now filled with hope and the belief that you can get better. I brought you to the Butterfly Mountain because it's a magical place filled with endless possibilities and the butterflies are here to encourage you to fly with all that you have learned. A new and exciting beginning is right in front of you – but you must grab it and enjoy it, with all the techniques you've learned on the journey there to help you. But the most important thing to remember is that the only person who can make this happen is *you*. Live it, breathe it every day. Keep focused on what you want and remember that where your focus goes, your energy flows.'

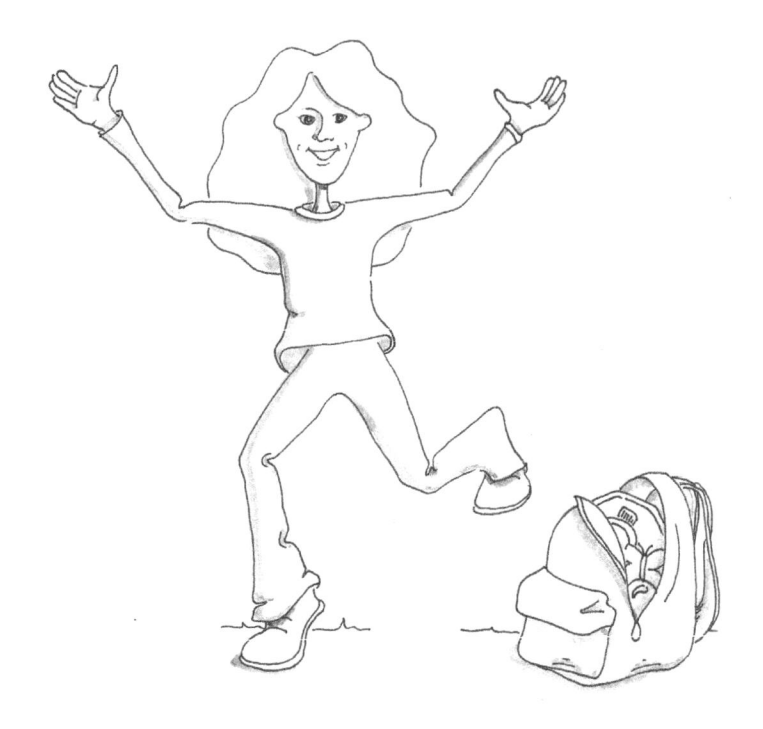

As I continue to gaze into the lake, I notice a golden bubble start to appear around me. It's as if someone is drawing it. I'm reminded of meeting Billie Bubble and the idea of the bubble protecting me, keeping those boundaries in place and being careful who and what I allow into this bubble. It's also a reminder of my environment, to whom and what I listen and speak. As the full circle is completed, Billie Bubble appears in the water as if they're reminding me never to forget. Billie's reflection slowly disappears and so too does the bubble around me.

As the picture in the lake becomes clearer, I realise I can see the faces of all the characters I've met on my journey.

They're all smiling. Then I hear Lexi barking loudly. I pull myself away from the vision and turn around. They're all standing right in front of me, each holding their canes with the symbols intact.

'You didn't think we'd miss out on saying goodbye to you, did you?' says Hugo.

Seeing them standing all together makes me feel quite emotional. They've all supported me on my journey and have taught me so much. I go over and hug each one of them.

'I want to thank you all from the bottom of my heart for equipping me with ways to manage my health. When I started out on this journey I felt completely lost with no control over my life. You've given me back control and helped me to feel empowered again by giving me knowledge. Knowledge is power! You've filled my toolkit with ideas and suggestions that will help me to move forward. Whatever circumstances are thrown at me I now feel I can cope. How wrong the GP was to tell me there's nothing I can do to help myself. I now know that I can bring myself out of the fight or flight response by doing breathing techniques.'

Barbara Bellows lifts her cane up high and gives me a huge smile.

'And If I find my mind is snowballing out of control or playing a tennis match with my thoughts, I can try the STOP technique. And that's great because I do that a lot!'

Clara Calm lifts her STOP symbol and I can't help but start singing one of my favourite songs, Meatloaf's 'Paradise by the Dashboard Light'. It isn't long before we're all singing and dancing. In fact, Henry Happy starts twirling me around. We soon collapse into a heap, laughing and full of happiness.

'Don't worry, Henry; I'll keep smiling even when I find it hard and just the corners of my mouth turn upwards. I'll start every day with a smile.'

Toby Time comes and sits beside me. 'You've done brilliantly to get to this point and you must feel so proud of yourself but to continue on this path you need to stick to your baseline. Don't overdo things or push yourself too hard – I know what you're like. As an achiever and a perfectionist, you'll drive yourself and end up back where you started. Be gentle and kind to yourself. Find your baseline and stick to it, then slowly move the baseline as you improve. If you do push yourself too hard one day and end up having a bit of a relapse, don't beat yourself up. Learn from it and move on. Don't overthink it. You can't undo what has been done but you can make new choices based on what you've learned. As you know, what you say to yourself is so important.'

I thank him as he holds up the watch on the top of his cane. And I'm still mesmerised by his piercing blue eyes!

'My focus will be making sure I'm careful to keep within my limits and not to do too much. However, I'm aware that my body needs to move – so, Milo, I'll be careful of my posture and try some yoga moves.'

Milo smiles and lifts his cane with the yoga figure on top. Then he puts it down, sits cross legged and brings his hands together near his heart. We all follow and enjoy this peaceful moment of feeling connected with ourselves and each other.

While we're all sitting in this relaxed state it makes me think of all the habits that Hana told me about. 'Hana, your ideas about forming good habits have really hit home. When I wake up in the morning, I'm going to smile then think of three things to be grateful for before doing some affirmations. Once I'm up and out of bed I will high five myself in the mirror just to remind myself of how awesome I am!'

'Don't forget the importance of getting out in nature,' says Hana as she lifts her cane up high, showing off the tree symbol on top.

'The tree reminds me of the importance of laying down good foundations so I can thrive and survive,' I tell her.

After a short while, Harpreet Health and Felicity Food both stand up. They start juggling different coloured pieces of fruit and vegetables! It's truly a sight to behold, especially when the fruit and veg come crashing down on top of them. It makes us all laugh.

'You two have made a huge impact on me,' I say, continuing to laugh. 'When I get home, I'm going to look in my food cupboard and fridge and think about which foods might be inflammatory and put me into the fight or flight response and those that will support my gut health and help me. The cans of cola will have to go. I'm beginning to appreciate that food is my medicine and will help me to heal. I promise to eat the rainbow and drink more water!'

Felicity lifts up her cane with its rainbow cup and beams at me.

'I'll also look after all my cells by giving them the food they need,' I continue. 'Harpreet, understanding that 70–80 per cent of my immune system lives in my gut will spur me on to look after it. I'm only as healthy as my gut.'

Harpreet lifts up her cane with GH on the top and says, 'You really have taken on board all we've said, which is fantastic. Now go and do it!'

'That's my plan.'

Next, I see Herbie Holistic holding up the fish symbol on his cane.

'I haven't forgotten you! The fish analogy is embedded in my mind. I'm going to look after all of my cells and my liver by looking after all of myself. I'll fill up my body with all the good stuff.'

Hugo Hope then looks at me and says, 'It's so good to hear your voice full of authority and belief. What a journey you have been on.' He lifts his cane with the butterfly on top.

I sit back and realise how tired I'm beginning to feel.

I hear a soft, gentle and familiar voice behind me. It's Nathan Night, holding up his cane with its moon symbol.

'To fully rest and repair you must sleep well,' he says.

'I now appreciate that sleep is my medicine too,' I tell him. 'I'm going to make sure I get off my phone and computer an hour before I go to bed and listen to a sleep meditation.'

'Close your eyes,' says Nathan.

I follow his instruction and feel him gently massaging the sides of my head. It's so soothing. I feel my breathing slow down and my mind relax. I'm soon drifting off to sleep.

After what seems like an eternity, I open my eyes and instead of Nathan Night, I see my dear friend Catherine. We're both sitting on the log where it all began.

'You just drifted off for a few minutes,' she says. 'You look different, though – you look more relaxed, more radiant. Are you OK?'

'I feel good, thanks. How long have I been asleep?'

'Oh, only about five minutes.'

I'm still holding my front door key – the one she returned. I slowly get up from the log, give her a huge hug and say that I will call her so we can catch up very soon.

I call Lexi and we start walking back home. But I feel different. I feel more positive – as if anything were possible. I put my hands in my pocket and my fingers wrap around something small and smooth. I take it out and stare at it. It's a marble. I wonder why it's there?

I arrive at my house and the first thing I notice is that my garden has been cleared of weeds and is looking loved and lovely. I feel so grateful to whoever has done this for me. I let Lexi and myself in and catch a glimpse of my reflection in the mirror. Catherine is right; I do look different. There's a definite glow around me and I do look much more relaxed. I go to the fridge to reach for a cola but stop myself. Something deep inside tells me to get a glass of filtered water instead. I shut the fridge, grab a drink of water and make some herbal tea. I open the cupboard to see what I'm going to eat tonight but quickly realise I should be making something with the vegetables I have in my fridge. 'What's going on?' I think to myself. 'It's as if my mind has been possessed!' But I look at the marble in my hand and wonder what else I'm going to discover. I'm excited and feel a real sense of hope. This is a new feeling and one I want to hold on to.

    I sit down on my favourite velvet green chair with my water and herbal tea and enjoy this new me. I pick up one of my favourite books, Charlie Mackesy's *The Boy, the Mole, the Fox and the Horse,* and it falls open at the page that says, 'One day you'll see how hard it was and how brave you were...'

CHAPTER 10

MAKING SENSE OF IT ALL

Time to look at you

I hope you've enjoyed travelling with Angela and Lexi on their magical journey. Here's a summary of all the characters they met along the way and what they represent:

Characters	What they stand for
Hugo Hope	Hope and keeping focus
Barbara Bellows	Breathing techniques
Billie Bubble	Protective bubble and environment
Henry Happy	Smile and be happy
Clara Calm	STOP technique
Toby Time	Baseline and pacing
Felicity Food	Food and drink – the 80:20 rule
Nathan Night	Sleep techniques
Hana Habit	Good morning habits
Milo Movement	Posture and yoga
Harpreet Health	Gut health
Herbie Holistic	The whole of you

Now, sit back and take a deep breath. I want you to take everything in slowly – there's no rush. You can pick up this book, put it down or re-read a chapter when you need to. It has taken me years to develop these techniques and there's nothing in this book that I haven't tried myself. These are just the basics for you to start with – a few ideas to play with.

Recovery isn't a straight upward trajectory – it has its highs and lows. But there's always hope. Don't forget to celebrate every day, however small that celebration might be. Remember that at the age of 27, I was celebrating just having a shower each morning. Your body is amazing. All it's trying to do is look after you, so thank it and love it regardless of how hard this may be. And at times I know it can feel really hard.

This chapter is about you, taking time to look at yourself and reflect on what you've read in the book so far. What has resonated with you? Remember: you're the only one who can make the changes. Immerse yourself in your recovery like the butterfly described in the introduction. Live and breathe it every single day but do it with kindness. Having read the book, what would you like to do today that may make a difference?

To help summarise everything I came up with the idea of the 3 Bs: **back to basics, being true to yourself** and **being brave**.

Back to basics

There are three key aspects to getting back to basics:

1. rest and repair versus fight or flight
2. the four basic needs of cells to survive and thrive
3. pacing and smiling.

Rest and repair versus fight or flight

Getting into the rest and repair response and out of the fight or flight one in all areas of my health, my mind and my body was so crucial for recovery that I want to stand up and shout it from the rooftops. This is what Hugo Hope talked about. As a useful exercise, think of three things you might be doing that are putting your body into the fight or flight response through your food, your thoughts or your environment. Then think of three things that you may be doing to put yourself into the rest and repair response.

Complete the table below or just think about it:

Fight or flight response	Rest and repair response
1	1
2	2
3	3

The four basic needs of cells to survive and thrive

- oxygen
- water
- elimination of waste
- nutrition.

We know that the mitochondria, the powerhouses that provide energy, are found in our cells and the key to a healthy body is having healthy cells. I'm sure you now know how many cells we have in our body as I've mentioned it a few times! I found that thinking about the body being made up of individual cells helped me to put my focus on each cell, helping me to recover. I could then begin to appreciate what these cells needed to survive.

Oxygen
The only way we can get oxygen into the body is by breathing it in. Barbara Bellows talked about this. I do breathing exercises first thing in the morning then throughout the day. If I feel myself coming into the fight or flight response, it helps me to rest and relax. It's simple but so effective. Milo Movement discussed yoga techniques, which help with breathing and movement, including bowel movements. Yoga helped me and still does. I also do the Wim Hof breathing techniques that you can find online (see resources section).

Water
I've mentioned water a lot in the book because it's so important to keep yourself hydrated. It helps to reduce the internal stress in your body. This is another point I want to shout from the rooftops! When I came down with CFS for the second time all I did for four months was to increase my water intake. Just doing this helped my energy. As Dr Batmanghelidj says in his 1992 book *Your Body's Many Cries for Water*, '... every function of the body is monitored and pegged to the efficient flow of water. "Water distribution" is the only way of making sure that not only an adequate amount of water, but its transported elements (hormones, chemical messengers and nutrients) first reach the more vital organs.' You can also increase your water through the food you eat. I make flaxseed tea daily and have lots of soups, smoothies and casseroles. I make flaxseed tea by putting two tablespoons of whole flaxseeds into a flask, adding boiling water, leaving it overnight to stew then drinking it throughout the next day. I eat cucumbers, celery, watermelon and spinach, which all have a high water content. I also try to avoid dehydrating foods such as crackers and rice cakes, and soak my legumes.

Which three things can you do to help with getting oxygen into your body? This may include some new breathing techniques or thinking about when you're going to do them during the day. Try setting a timer on your phone. You could also go to a breathwork practitioner to help and guide you.

Which three things can help you hydrate? Are you going to buy a new water bottle, a water filter or make some flaxseed tea? Fill in the table below to help guide you.

Getting oxygen in	Increasing hydration
1.	1.
2.	2.
3.	3.

Elimination of waste

The third point is the elimination of waste. You don't want to hold onto toxins as that will create havoc in your body. Aim to have a good bowel movement every day, as Harpreet Health suggested. I continue to work on this daily and am aware of how important it is. Herbie Holistic also talked about eliminating toxins from the body through breathing, urination and the skin. Be careful which creams you put on your skin; let it breathe. Having a sauna also helps to remove toxins. I used to sit in a sauna for 20 minutes a couple of times a week, especially when my energy was low. Also look after your lovely liver.

Nutrition

The final point is nutrition. Your body is only as healthy as the food you put into it. This was a profound realisation for me. I thought I ate well but hadn't truly connected with the fact that what you put into your mouth creates you – new skin, hair, cells, mitochondria, cell membranes, protein, hormones, etc. It's important to remove foods that may cause inflammation in the body such as sugar and processed or refined foods. Also, replacing drinks that act as stimulants, such as tea, coffee and alcohol, with herbal teas and decaffeinated coffee. If possible, eat the rainbow and organic and unrefined foods.

Felicity Food and Herbie Holistic talked about the good fats we need for our cell membranes but also for our skin, digestion, brain function, etc. Using olive oil and coconut oil and eating food containing omega-3 such as flaxseed, chia seeds, avocados and walnuts is important. You can put yourself into the rest and repair response through the food and drink you consume but also important are how you eat it and the mindset you're in when you do so. Harpreet Health discussed food and the importance of gut health. She also discussed prebiotic and probiotic foods. Small changes can have a huge impact on you. Gut health is crucial for long-term recovery.

Dr Sarah Myhill, who has spent her medical life treating patients with CFS, stresses the importance of cutting out gluten or dairy. This alone stopped my bloating and once I increased my water, fibre and good fats, my bowels functioned brilliantly. As Dr Will Bulsiewicz says in his 2020 book *Fibre Fuelled*, 'Nobody is talking about boring old fibre. I am here to tell you that fibre is the first and potentially the most powerful solution to restoring health to your gut microbiome and from there overall health.' There's a four-week diet plan at the back of the book, which I followed. It may not be for everyone but I found it helpful.

Which three things could you do to help with the removal of waste from your body? You could hydrate, increase your fibre intake through fruit and vegetables, go to the sauna or look at the products you are using on your skin to allow it to breathe.

Which three things are you going to add to your diet? Are you going to increase your fruit and vegetables? If so, which ones might you try this week? Maybe try some different grains such as brown rice, wholemeal pasta, quinoa or buckwheat. What about having some omega-3s in your diet? How about trying some nuts and seeds? Maybe look at trying olive oil and coconut oil. Are there any probiotics you can try, such as sauerkraut or miso?

Removal of waste	Food and drink to add to your diet
1	1
2	2
3	3

Pacing and smiling

As Toby Time discussed, back to basics also includes pacing yourself. This is crucial for recovery and stops you putting your body into the fight or flight response. When I learned about pacing, it was a lightbulb moment. I've had many of those on my recovery journey but this was like a chandelier! Find your baseline and stick to it. If you push too hard too soon, you'll crash and get frustrated and fed up. I know that feeling only too well. I started to make progress once I discovered the importance of sticking to my baseline. It wasn't easy, believe me. As an achiever, holding back was hard and it wasn't until I truly stuck to it that I started to make big improvements. Remember the hare and the tortoise story? Slow and steady wins the race.

The last point in this section relates to Henry Happy. Is it easy to smile and be happy when you feel awful? No, of course it's not but it's the message you send to yourself that's important. I woke up every morning, tuned into myself and my mind and then smiled. Whatever the day brought, this helped. Watch films that make you giggle or a comedy sketch, or have a laugh with friends. I did a lot of this, which helped to lift my spirits. When I was able to go for a walk, I'd smile the whole way, trying to be in the moment.

A few years ago I came across a Buddhist monk from Vietnam called Thich Nhat Hanh, who was once nominated for a Nobel Peace Prize. He really touched my heart and soul. His little book called *Peace Is Every Step* (1991) was a huge influence on me. I'd only look at a page at a time. I didn't have the energy to read more but everything I did read was so beautiful and helped me to think about things differently. For example, he writes, 'If you have lost your smile and yet are still capable of seeing that a dandelion is keeping it for you then the situation is not too bad.' I loved this because at that stage I didn't have the capacity to smile – I felt too sad. How gorgeous is that?

Do you need to think about your own pacing? Are you pushing yourself in certain areas that you need to look at? Which three things could you do to help slow yourself down? Do you need more smiling and laughter in your life? I certainly did. How are you going to do this? Which three things make you smile – family, friends, a film, a comedian, a memory, sunshine?

Pacing	Smile
1.	1.
2.	2.
3.	3.

Being true to yourself

This means looking at the mind–body connection. The vagus nerve, which connects these two, is like a housekeeper, keeping everything in order. The mind is so powerful. I've been on a steep learning curve and there have been times when I doubted what I was reading and listening to. It wasn't until I started applying it all myself that I grasped the concepts.

In 2022, I listened to Dr Rangan Chatterjee interview developmental biologist Bruce Lipton on his podcast *Feel Better Live More*. I was reminded that your behaviour is based on your beliefs, which you inherited when you were young so that you could receive love and stay safe. You play up to these beliefs throughout your life, even after you've stopped needing them – beliefs such as 'I'm not worthy', 'I'm not good enough' or 'I feel powerless'. 'I'm not good enough' is one of mine. These beliefs were stopping me from making a full recovery and I know they've had an impact on many people's recovery journeys. Acknowledging these beliefs but *not* allowing them to have power, then creating new ones that suit you better, is transformative. You have the power to change them – this is so important.

You may be thinking, 'How do I reprogram my beliefs?' Bruce Lipton suggests three ways of doing this. The first is about forming habits, as Hana Habit discussed. Angela learned about the importance of getting into good daily habits so that they become automatic. It's like learning to drive. At first it all seems too difficult – you have to break down each process but after a while you just get into a car and drive because you've done it so many times. So when you're having a bad day and your habits have become automatic you'll just carry them out. This can have a profound effect on you and your mindset. I have practised habits daily but I've changed them depending on what I felt I needed at the time.

My daughter gave me a book by James Clear called *Atomic Habits* (2018). It talks about how changing small things every day can have a huge impact but that transformation can be slow and therefore bad habits can slide back in. A slight change in habit can guide your life to a very different destination. I love his analogy of a plane. If the pilot is flying from Los Angeles to New York City and adjusts the route by 3.5 degrees south, the plane will land in Washington. When the plane takes off it's barely noticeable but over a larger distance it ends up hundreds of miles away. Stick with it – don't give up, be kind to yourself and ask for help.

The second way to reprogram involves the hypnotic state that you experience just as you fall asleep. In this state your subconscious mind kicks in. This is a great time to listen to a meditation, a recording of what you want or a self-help programme. Your subconscious will take it in and remember it. Nathan Night did a sleep meditation and discussed a few ideas that might help with your sleep. Believe me, I've tried them all. The third way is by using 'energy psychology', which you'll need to do with a practitioner (see the recommended resources at the end). They will help you engage the subconscious and reprogram your thought patterns. I've done this myself and it was a powerful experience.

At the start of the book, Angela finds out she has CFS and is told by her GP that there's nothing more that can be done for her. She goes on to discover that there are things she can do that give her back some power. She takes back control of her life by changing her mindset and beliefs. Which three things do you do already that help you to form habits such as gratitudes, high fives, meditation, mindfulness, walking outside in nature, breathwork, exercise or sleep routine? Is there anything you need to add, such as looking at your beliefs, your mindset or anything else I've mentioned?

You may want to write three things down but just start with one if you want to.

Habits I already have	New ideas to look at
1.	1.
2.	2.
3.	3.

Toby Morris from CFS Health talks about three key essentials that you must have to recover.

The first is behaviour. Having a set of behaviours to help with recovery is vital. He says that you can't move forward with the same behaviours that got you to crash in the first place. For example, I was an achiever and a helper and would help others before helping myself. Toby Time talked about being an achiever and Clara Calm discussed the STOP technique, which helps to change your thought patterns and behaviour by changing your focus. I used to walk the dog and when I had a negative thought that would snowball, I'd shout 'STOP' at the top of my voice, regardless of who was listening! If nothing else, it always made me smile.

The second is your belief system. Toby explained that what you're telling yourself is so important. Do you believe you'll make a complete recovery? It wasn't until I looked at my mindset that I turned a huge corner. This included visualising myself fully recovered, seeing and believing it, because up to that point, I don't think I truly believed I'd get better.

The third is your environment. What and who are you surrounding yourself with daily? Billie Bubble talks about forming a bubble to protect yourself. Having this bubble helped me stay true to myself and hold off other people's thoughts, views and opinions that didn't resonate with me. If you have a good environment, one that's positive and uplifting, this will shape your behaviour and hence your beliefs. While I was lying down for most of the day, I listened to podcasts, followed people who inspired me, watched films I'd been meaning to watch for ages and listened to audiobooks when reading was too much of an effort. I watched a lot of romcoms!

Which behaviours do you think led you to where you are now? Which behaviours influenced your energy levels? Do you need to look at your achiever pattern? Are you too much of a helper, giving all your energy to others? What are you telling yourself daily? Do you need to think about your environment – who you talk to, give your energy to and how long you're talking to them? What are you listening to and watching? Is there a new podcast you might listen to, a film to watch, a book to read, a course to go on, a new person to follow on a social media platform?

Fill in the table below or just think about it.

My behaviour/beliefs	My environment
1.	1.
2.	2.
3.	3.

Being brave

Why am I putting an emphasis on being brave? Because it's important. It's hard to deal with CFS or long Covid. Others may not understand and you'll be trying to explain complex symptoms that vary from day to day. Being brave is tough but necessary on a recovery journey. Days can feel long and challenging and you'll feel lost and sad. Hugo Hope believed in Angela. He encouraged her to be brave and focus on what she wanted, to get to the Butterfly Mountain and not give up. As I say throughout the book, 'Where your focus goes, your energy flows.' Focus on what you want, whether that's your end goal or a daily objective. In Charlie Mackesy's book, the boy says he sometimes feels he hasn't done much. Then the horse says, 'You've got up and carried on... which is brave and magnificent.' When I read this, I thought to myself, 'Yup, that's me, I'm brave and magnificent.' I've carried on after being knocked down numerous times. I loved this as it helped me to feel proud of myself. Asking for help is a brave thing to do because you have to acknowledge you're struggling and show vulnerability. I found this hard to do at first. Think of Angela. At the beginning she ignored her friend Catherine's phone calls. She didn't want to talk to her even though Catherine was only checking up on her. But in Chapter 9, she eventually did. Humans need connection, even if it's only a ten-minute phone call or visit.

A few years ago, a group of friends suggested I watched Brené Brown's TED talk on the power of vulnerability. I remember thinking, 'Why on earth would I want to watch that? This isn't what I need right now.' But I was wrong. Brown talks about connection being the reason we're here; as she says, 'The ability to feel connected is how we are wired.' Even though it may feel hard to do, talking to family and friends will stop you from feeling disconnected.

Being brave is also about making tough choices on your recovery journey. For instance, saying no to things that you'd like to do to help yourself with your pacing, smiling when you don't feel like it, carrying out daily habits when you're just not in the mood. But recovery is about showing up every day with this intention – living and breathing it so you'll believe it. As Herbie Holistic said, looking at the whole of you is crucial. Most importantly, love yourself, which is brave when you feel so rough.

Learning to truly love yourself can be a journey of its own but is so worthwhile. I found this particularly challenging but so impactful for my recovery journey. By loving myself I was loving every cell in my body.

Which three things are you being brave about now that need celebrating?

Three things I'm being brave about that need celebrating
1.
2.
3.

I hope this conclusion helps you to understand why Angela went on her journey and how it was inspired by my own. If you're wondering how I'm doing now – thank you for asking! As I said in the introduction, when I first went down with CFS I was rowing and working as a physiotherapist. I can't believe that I'm now rowing again after 25 years away from a boat. I'm loving it – and I have my own business as well. I've come a long way over the past few years but I wouldn't have been able to do it without hope, determination and being tough about my decisions. I'm still making those tough decisions now. I must still be careful and monitor what I'm doing but I have a huge toolkit that I can dip into when necessary. I also have family and friends who keep tabs on me and give me gentle nudges when I default to some of my unhelpful habits.

Of course, there are other things you can do but start with the basics, get these right and then build on them. For instance, you may need more tests or supplements but the ideas in this book will work well alongside other treatments. Remember to set your own goals, however small or big. They are *your* goals because you're the only one who can make the changes. Own them. Set an intention of what you really want to do now, commit to it, then visualise it and hold it in your mind. Visualisation is extremely powerful. But how are you going to make sure you stay on track? Are you going to keep a journal, record it on your phone, use an app, tell someone, take photos, draw? Whatever it is, hold yourself to it. Make yourself accountable. Tell yourself what you want and when you wake up every morning, picture it. To whoever is reading this book: you can draw on all your strengths to help you to recover. Use them! You've got this.

I want to wish you well on your healing journey. Know that I understand what you're going through. I want to give each one of you a magic marble. Hold on to it tightly and let it remind you of Angela's mission. I hope you now have a few tools in your toolkit. I'm sure you'll need more but they'll give you a start – a great start.

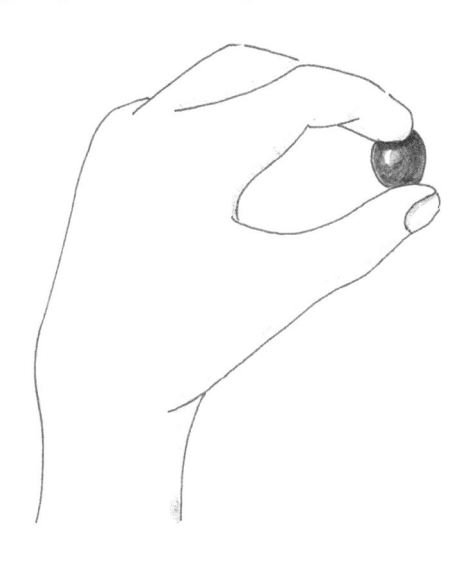

BACK IN THE REAL WORLD

THE RESOURCES SECTION

Explaining the why and how

This section explains more about what you've been introduced to in each chapter of Angela's story. This information is here for you when you have more energy to absorb it. Don't read on until you're up to it. At the end of the section there's a list of helpful websites, articles, books, podcasts and TED talks.

Introduction
What exactly is CFS?
Here are the facts. The National Institute for Health and Care Excellence (NICE) guidelines state that 'ME/CFS can affect people of all ages. It is a complex, multi-system, chronic medical condition that has considerable personal, social and economic consequences and a significant impact on a person's quality of life, including their psychological, emotional and social wellbeing.' It goes on to say, 'Recent data from the UK Biobank… suggest that there are over 250,000 people in England and Wales with ME/CFS, with about 2.4 times as many women affected as men.'

The ME Association says that CFS should be suspected if a person has had all four of the key symptoms for a minimum of six weeks in adults and four weeks in children. There's a huge amount of information on their website but the four key symptoms are:

- debilitating fatigue that is worsened by activity
- post-exertional malaise/symptom exacerbation
- unrefreshing sleep or sleep disturbance
- cognitive dysfunction.

Why do people get CFS or long Covid?
Just like every snowflake is different, every human being is unique. You can't compare yourself to anyone else and when thinking about why you may have one of these conditions, don't be judgemental; just acknowledge it. I believe it starts before you're born – it's part of your genetic make-up, what you've inherited. Then it depends on what has happened in your life, starting with any childhood illnesses and how they were treated. Which physical or emotional traumas and stresses have occurred in your life? Which food and drink has impacted your gut health and immune system? Have you been exposed to any toxins and how good is your body at getting rid of these? Have you had any viruses or bacterial infections? How about Lyme disease? Or food poisoning?

Some people with CFS have problems converting fuel into energy. It can occur at any age but mainly in young to middle-aged adults. Some may have other underlying medical issues. Your mindset is important as well. What's your environment like? Do you truly believe you will recover? Your personality type may also play a part. For example, do you push and drive yourself hard? Are you always on the go with no time to let your body rest and repair? What's your sleep like? I could go on but I hope you get the picture. Hopefully you'll now have an idea as to why you have one of these conditions.

Why did I get CFS/long Covid?
I believe it was because I took a lot of antibiotics at a young age. I had tonsilitis and later glandular fever, which is caused by the Epstein-Barr virus and can be a precursor to

CFS. Also, the first time I had CFS, I'd been driving myself hard. I had a physical job as a physiotherapist, I was rowing and training five times a week as well as doing a postgrad course. I also had a full social life. I didn't stop and my body had no time to rest and recover. The second time I crashed was different. It was both physical and emotional. I'd been pushing myself on my road bike, climbing mountains in Majorca; we'd moved house and location; the kids had changed schools; I'd changed jobs; and then I had a hysterectomy. Now, you may be thinking that's a lot – and it was. But shortly afterwards my mum died. She was my rock and I crumbled. I was a wreck. I felt as if one of the legs on a three-legged stool had been removed and my solid base had collapsed. It wasn't long after this that I went down with CFS for the second time. Later, when I had long Covid, I think it was because of everything that my body had been through and my immune system was low. But in that instance, due to all the tools I had in my toolbox, I did recover well.

Chapter 1
The fight or flight and the rest and repair responses

The best way to describe these responses is through the scenario of a zebra being chased by a lion. The lion is charging through the grassy plains of Africa in pursuit of the zebra. In that moment all the zebra's energy needs to be focused on survival and escaping from the lion. The zebra is in the fight or flight response, which releases bursts of hormones such as adrenaline. How does the zebra divert its energy to respond to the danger? Blood is diverted to its muscles to help it to run and to its heart and lungs to increase its breathing rate and heart rate. It doesn't need to waste energy on digestion, excretion or the immune system so none of these systems work efficiently during the fight or flight response. The zebra survives and can then think about what it's going to eat for breakfast.

It's living in the moment; it doesn't think about yesterday or tomorrow and, if necessary, can quickly switch from fight or flight into rest and repair. The zebra's heart rate and breathing rate drop, it finds a lovely patch of luscious grass and it starts eating. It's now calm and can focus on digesting the grass, repairing, excreting and letting the immune system do its work. The rest and repair response has now been triggered.

The key point is that the zebra can't be in both responses at the same time. It can either relax and eat the grass and let its body rest and repair and digest or be in the fight or flight response, running from the lion. It's the same with your body. When it's in the stress response it can't digest properly, sleep, excrete or allow the immune system to work efficiently because it's responding to 'danger'. This can be stress, your thoughts or what you eat and drink as well as physical activity. The zebra is good at switching from fight or flight to rest and repair but most humans stay in the stress response due to overthinking about what happened yesterday, what could have happened and what may happen tomorrow rather than just being in the moment. When this occurs, it can lead to chronic stress, mood changes, adrenal fatigue, difficulty sleeping, irritable bowel syndrome, chronic inflammation and other health issues. Understanding how to keep out of this response by saving energy and diverting it to where it's needed is crucial to recovery.

These responses are part of the nervous system, which is made up of an amazing network of nerves that covers your whole body. According to Healthline, these 'act in different functions to keep your body moving, responding, sensing and more'. The sympathetic nervous system (SNS) triggers the fight or flight response. The rest and repair or rest and digest response is also known as the parasympathetic nervous system (PNS), which conserves energy and maintains the vital bodily functions mentioned above. The

Resources

SNS and PNS are part of the autonomic nervous system (ANS). The ANS is the part of the nervous system that you have no control over. It just gets on with its job of looking after you, outside your conscious control.

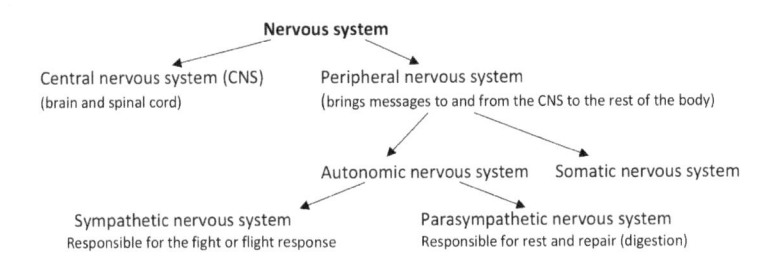

```
                         Nervous system
                        ↙            ↘
Central nervous system (CNS)    Peripheral nervous system
(brain and spinal cord)         (brings messages to and from the CNS to the rest of the body)
                                       ↙            ↘
                          Autonomic nervous system    Somatic nervous system
                         ↙              ↘
Sympathetic nervous system         Parasympathetic nervous system
Responsible for the fight or flight response   Responsible for rest and repair (digestion)
```

Chapter 2
Breathing techniques

Angela was taught the 4-7-8 breathing technique, which can help you to relax and stimulates your parasympathetic nervous system – the rest and repair response. It's also known as the 'relaxation breath' and has ancient roots in pranayama, which is the yogic practice of breath regulation. This is why yoga can be so helpful, just for the breathwork alone. This technique also helps to regulate the hormone cortisol, which controls the fight or flight response. It can also help with sleep as it relaxes the mind and helps to reduce anxiety and stress. But you need to start slowly, repeating it only three or four times until you get used to it. There is also the 4-6 technique that immediately changes your focus and keeps you calm. It is easier to do and a great one to start off with if you have never done any breathwork before. And there's the Wim Hof method, which is a breathing technique that helps to release more energy, influences your nervous system, helps you mentally and physiologically and helps you feel more in control. I've used this technique and it's very powerful.

Your beliefs – the helper type

Delving into my beliefs was a lightbulb moment for me. You inherit many of your beliefs in order to get your needs met – mostly love and safety. In his book *The Biology of Belief* (2015) Bruce Lipton says, 'Learning how to harness your mind to promote growth is the secret of life.' He goes on to say, 'Your genes do not dictate your life and you can change your life when you change your beliefs.' Lipton, a cell biologist by training, is an internationally recognised leader in bridging science and spirit.

Many people with CFS are natural helpers who give their time and energy to others, so they have nothing left for themselves. If you're a helper type, then you'll have learned from a young age that to be safe and accepted you must look after everyone else. Helper types often go on to be part of the helping profession and try hard to keep everyone happy and not let others down. As I learned on the 90-day programme at the Optimum Health Clinic, they will often 'subjugate their own needs to be there for others... they will often feel unsupported and even angry with those around them... eventually the body must find a way to stop us and force us to look after ourselves'.

Your environment

As I explained at the end of this chapter, your environment is important: what you listen to, what you watch and who you talk to will directly correlate with your beliefs and behaviour. It will also have an impact on your energy levels. If you don't have much of it, be careful who you give your energy to. When I was at the start of my recovery, I had a weekly calendar (kindly given to me) that I'd fill in each day. I'd write down everything I was going to do and that included seeing or talking to people. I had limited energy, so I'd only talk for a few minutes or see someone for ten minutes and I'd be careful who I saw or spoke to. You have that control. It wasn't until I truly believed I'd recover and that I alone held that key that things really started to improve.

Smiling
This is so simple but can have a big impact on the body. Smiling can help to reduce stress and boost your immune system by reducing cortisol levels. When you smile your body releases endorphins and serotonin, creating positive emotions.

Chapter 3
Sunshine, vitamin D and serotonin
Sunlight is our main source of vitamin D and we make around 90 per cent of it through our skin. Vitamin D also helps with the production of serotonin, which impacts our mood, sleep and appetite. Serotonin is our happy hormone. It can also affect sleep as serotonin helps to produce melatonin, which is a hormone that helps to prepare your body for sleep. Exposing your skin to sunshine for 15 to 30 minutes a day will provide most of the vitamin D you need, except maybe in winter. Vitamin D is necessary for the absorption of calcium and phosphorus, which are required to keep bones, teeth and muscles healthy. You may need a supplement throughout the autumn and winter, as the sun won't be strong enough to produce enough vitamin D. I take vitamin D with magnesium because it helps with absorption but do discuss this with your nutritionist or GP.

Being in nature
Being in nature is associated with better health and wellbeing. It can help with anxiety and stress and impacts your mood, helping you to feel more relaxed. According to an article on the American Psychological Association's website (2020), 'There is so much evidence from research that nature has benefits for both physical and physiological human wellbeing.'

It has been suggested that if you hug a tree for a minimum of 20 seconds, oxytocin (the feel-good hormone) is released in your body and brings many benefits. It can be the same if you hug another person. It helps to boost the immune system, reduces stress and gives you a feeling of connection. Give it a go – if nothing else it will make you smile or laugh. I love it. I now rest my ear against the tree as I hug it and just let myself breathe and listen.

The STOP technique
This is a mindfulness technique designed to help you defuse stress in the moment. It can also be called the STOPP technique, with the additional P standing for plan. Plan what you're going to do next. What's the most important thing for you to do now? P can also stand for practise – practise this method repeatedly so that it comes easily to you.

The vagus nerve
This helps to counteract the fight or flight response and put you into the rest and repair state by helping you to stay calm. You can stimulate the vagus nerve by doing such things as singing or even gargling. This helps the immune system as well as the inflammatory response to disease. The vagus nerve is the longest cranial nerve, connecting the brain stem to the body. It sends information from your gut to the brain and vice versa, which is why your gut health is so important.

Pacing and keeping to a baseline
According to naturopathic physician Dr Sarah Myhill in her book *Diagnosis and Treatment of Chronic Fatigue Syndrome and Myalgic Encephalitis* (2017), 'Pacing and rest are vital in CFS to start the process of recovery and ensure the continuation of such a recovery… Thinking of energy as money is very useful. CFS sufferers should always aim to have some money left at the end of the day so that their

bodies can spend this energy on recovery.' In Angela's story, money is replaced by marbles.

According to Action for ME, 'Baseline is a level of activity that you can sustain on a regular basis. In other words, you should be able to do the same baseline amount of activity day after day. Your baseline activity will be below your "personal best" that you can manage on a better day.' A podcast by CFS Health explains this further (see the list of useful podcast episodes at the end of this section).

Pacing is a self-management technique. The NICE guidelines call it 'energy management', which is a 'self-management strategy that involves a person with ME/CFS managing their activities to stay within their energy limit, with support from a health care professional'.

And the CFS Health website says, 'It can be so important to get to grips with the baseline as it can make a massive difference for long-term progress. It is sticking to it consistently which leads to progress… If you push and crash, nothing will work. So your baseline is being able to do what you can do without feeling any worse than you currently do.'

The achiever personality type
This is often typical of people with CFS. As an achiever you'll learn from an early age that to be accepted and loved you need to achieve and succeed. This is because your core belief is that you're not good enough so have to keep overachieving and pushing yourself, which leads to burnout. It's exhausting – but the good news is that once you recognise the pattern, you can let it go because the beliefs are no longer necessary. You can't get rid of them but you can strip them of their power by changing your focus. You can then set new beliefs and boundaries. The 90-day psychology programme I went through at the Optimum Health Clinic helped me to understand about beliefs and how to move on (as did reading books by Tony Robbins, William Whitecloud and Bruce Lipton).

Chapter 4

Whatever you put in your mouth, your body must deal with. Remember that food is your medicine but make changes slowly and without judgement. Do it with knowledge and be gentle with yourself. To remind you, the only change I made for four months was an increase in my water consumption. I made the other changes slowly and mindfully. Keep in mind the 80:20 rule.

Here's the chart that Felicity Food gave Angela:

Protein	Healthy fats	Carbohydrates	Fibre
Eggs, particularly egg white	Eggs	Wholegrains – brown rice, oats	Wholegrains – brown rice, oats
Nut and seeds – almonds and pumpkin seeds	Nuts – such as almonds, macadamia, walnuts	Vegetables such as peas, sweet potato, butternut squash	Vegetables such as peas, kale, cabbage, carrots
Poultry – chicken and turkey; red meat, such as grass-fed beef	Seeds such as chia, pumpkin, flax	Fruit such as mangos, bananas, apples	Fruit such as mangos, bananas, apples
Fish, such as salmon and cod	Fatty fish, such as salmon, mackerel and herring	Beans such as kidney beans, black beans and cannellini beans	Nuts such as pine nuts, almonds, walnuts
Soy products, eg tofu, tempeh and edamame	Avocados	Chickpeas	Pulses – tinned or dried, beans, lentils
Dairy products – milk, yoghurt and cheese	Dairy products – yoghurt and cheese	Dairy products – milk and yoghurt	Seeds, eg sesame, sunflower, flax and chia
Beans and legumes – black beans, lentils and chickpeas	Olive oil and coconut oil	Legumes such as lentils	

Sugar

The body needs glucose (sugar) to produce energy in the form of adenosine triphosphate (ATP), preferably from sugar in its natural state through fruit, vegetables and grains. A sharp increase in sugar from processed sugars will cause a rise in glucose levels in the bloodstream and will be followed by a crash. When your blood sugar spikes, your brain will 'panic' because it needs more glucose to keep running, so it pushes you into the flight or fight response and cues the adrenal glands to release the stress hormone cortisol, which signals you to eat more sugar. Stress leads you to reach for more sugar, which keeps you locked into the stress response and keeps you in fight or flight.

If sugar is consumed in the wrong form, it can create inflammation in the gut. You need your gut to be healthy because 70–80 per cent of the immune system is in there. Sugar molecules are classified as monosaccharides (such as glucose and fructose) and disaccharides (such as sucrose and lactose). A monosaccharide is a single sugar molecule. A disaccharide contains two monosaccharides. Fruit contains natural sugars, which are a mix of sucrose, glucose and fructose. Fructose is harmful but only in excessive amounts and not when it comes from fruit. When buying food, always check the label as many items contain hidden sugars such as fructose. Fructose in fruit is mixed with fibre, minerals and vitamins, which help with absorption in the gut. It would be difficult to eat excess fructose just by eating fruit.

In his book *Get Off Your Sugar* (2021), Daryl Gioffre says, 'A review of numerous studies published in the Mayo Clinic Proceedings in 2015 concluded that one type of sugar – fructose – is harder on your body. The digestive tract can't absorb it as well as it can glucose, sucrose, and other forms of sugar, meaning more of it gets sent to your liver where it contributes to a whole host of chronic illnesses.'

Water

Staying hydrated is important as it helps remove toxins and prevents dehydration. Water is crucial to your body and your health. As Dr Batmanghelidj says, 'The simple truth is that dehydration can cause diseases.' (1992) After all, we're made up of 70 per cent water. It's crucial for many things, including your digestion, cells, the removal of waste out of your body and the reduction of stress. I have a jug of filtered water in my kitchen. I take a pint of water to bed each night and as soon as I wake up, I drink the pint 30 minutes before breakfast. I then drink up to four pints throughout the day but never more than one pint in any hour. Using a water filter helps to remove the contaminants from drinking water.

Why is it important to eat the rainbow?

'Eat the rainbow' is the term used to describe colourful, plant-based food containing phytochemicals such as fruits, vegetables, wholegrains, nuts, seeds and legumes. Phytochemicals give plants their colour, flavour and aroma and have many health benefits. For instance, orange-coloured fruit and vegetables – carrots, sweet potatoes and pumpkins – contain the phytochemical beta-carotene, which helps to support healthy skin, eyes and the immune system. Eating the rainbow will give you a range of health benefits. It's better if you can eat organic, locally sourced, seasonal fruit and vegetables but don't worry if you can't.

Antioxidants

Some fruit and vegetables provide antioxidants such as vitamins C and E and carotenoids, which will support your recovery. Antioxidants are molecules that help to fight free radicals in your body and prevent many chronic diseases. Free radicals are a type of unstable molecule made during normal cell metabolism (chemical changes that take place in a cell). They're only dangerous when there are too many of them, because they can damage cells and are linked to a host of diseases. Foods high in free radicals include refined sugars and processed meats. Heating fats and oils such as vegetable oil to a high temperature also creates free radicals. Preservatives used in processed meats, including sausages, bacon, ham, pepperoni, hot dogs, salami, corned beef and many deli meats may also create free radicals.

Foods high in vitamin C	Foods high in vitamin E
Oranges, lemon, kiwi fruit	Spinach
Strawberries, blueberries	Sunflower seeds
Bell peppers	Avocados
Broccoli, brussels sprouts	Butternut squash
Cabbage, cauliflower	Leafy greens

Fats

There are three main types: saturated fats, unsaturated fats and trans fats. All fats are made up of carbon, hydrogen and oxygen molecules. Saturated fats are saturated with hydrogen molecules and contain only single bonds between carbon molecules. They are solid at room temperature. Unsaturated fats have at least one double between carbon molecules and are liquid at room temperature. Saturated fats are naturally occurring fats found in meat and dairy and are likely to be stored as fat, so choose them carefully – eat organic as much as possible and from trustworthy sources, especially when it comes to meat, fish and eggs. Saturated fats are also found in butter, lard, cakes, biscuits and pies. Most adults have too much saturated fat. Try to buy butter from organic, grass-fed cows.

Unsaturated fats are divided into two types – monounsaturated and polyunsaturated. Polyunsaturated fats include omega-3 and omega-6, which are essential fatty acids (EFAs) that can't be made by the body, which is why they're essential. EFAs are needed to make hormones, nourish our cells, feed our nerves and make neurotransmitters that send messages throughout our body. EFAs are also highly anti-inflammatory. A diet high in omega-3 helps with heart health, metabolism and immunity. They come from foods such as flaxseeds, fish, chia seeds and walnuts. If you eat fish, have oily fish such as salmon, trout and mackerel twice a week. Fats are easily damaged through exposure to light, heat and oxygen so go for oils that are cold compressed, which means they've been produced by natural methods.

Good monounsaturated fats are found in olives, avocados, nuts and seeds such as almonds, Brazil nuts, pine nuts, sesame seeds, peanuts and nut butters such as almond nut butter, which I use in smoothies and porridge. Trans fats (or hydrogenated fats) are found in two forms – natural or artificial. Artificial trans fats are hazardous to your health and can be found in margarine, cake mixes, and processed and fried foods. Like sugar, trans fats promote inflammation in the body, which can worsen your CFS signs and symptoms. These fats have been heavily processed to give them a longer shelf life, so try to eliminate oils such as sunflower oil and vegetable oil.

Saturated fats Limit these	Unsaturated fats Monounsaturated (M) Polyunsaturated (P) Eat lots of these!	Trans fats Reduce or avoid or bin!
Fats found in meat	M – olives, avocados, olive oil	Vegetable oil
Fats found in dairy such as butter, lard	M – Brazil nuts, pine nuts, sesame seeds, nut butters P – flaxseeds, chia seeds, walnuts	Margarine Non-dairy coffee creamer
Cakes, biscuits	P – oily fish	Food such as chips that have been fried in vegetable oil

Resources

Good fats are vital for your body and are an important part of a healthy balanced diet. Every cell has a double membrane that's full of fat. A cell membrane will only be as good as the fats that you consume, so eat healthy fats. You also need them to help you absorb fat-soluble vitamins – A, D, E and K. Most studies show that replacing saturated fats with unsaturated fats is a good idea.

Chapter 5

Sleep is crucial for recovery but when you're struggling with CFS it can take time to get a full night's sleep. Getting into the rest and repair state really can help. As Dr Sarah Myhill says in her book (2017), 'You must put as much effort into your sleep as diet. Without a good night's sleep on a regular basis, all other interventions are undermined.'

What is blue light?
Natural light contains a spectrum of colours, one of which is blue light. You need natural blue light during the day to stay awake and alert but you don't want it at night when you're trying to go to sleep. You have a natural circadian rhythm, which is the body's own biological clock. Your body wants to wake up when the sun rises and go to bed when the sun sets. Using artificial light after dark throws this circadian rhythm out of sync. Exposure to artificial light suppresses the secretion of the hormone melatonin, the sleep inducer. According to Stephen Lockley, a Harvard sleep researcher, light at night is part of the reason so many people don't get enough sleep. All light can suppress melatonin but blue light at night is the most powerful one. Computer screens, laptops, flatscreen TVs, mobile phones and tablets all emit blue light, so avoid using electronic devices before going to bed. The National Sleep Foundation suggests least 30 minutes before lights out. If you must use a computer or device, buy some glasses that block the blue light.

Magnesium salts
Having a warm bath with magnesium salts can help with relaxation before going to bed. Magnesium is often referred to as 'the natural tranquilliser' because of its calming, de-stressing effects. It helps stimulate the gamma-aminobutyric acid (GABA) receptors in the brain. According to Healthline (2021), 'GABA is the neurotransmitter responsible for quieting down activity. It is the same neurotransmitter used by sleep drugs. By helping to quiet the nervous system, magnesium may help to prepare your body and mind for sleep.'

Meditation for sleep
This can help in so many ways. It increases your natural melatonin levels, which help you get to sleep and feel calm and relaxed, putting you into the rest and repair state. There are endless free meditations available online and in various apps. I can recommend Linda Hall's meditations as well as Headspace (see the listings at the end of this section), which says that meditation 'helps to lower the heart rate by igniting the PNS and encouraging slower breathing'. To start with, I did ten minutes then built it up. I didn't find it easy to switch off at the beginning. My mind was struggling to let go and I had so much internal chatter but the more I practised the easier it became. Eventually I could meditate for an hour.

Chapter 6
Gratitude
According to Brain Balance, 'Gratitude can boost the neurotransmitter serotonin and activate the brain stem to produce dopamine.' Serotonin is the happy hormone and dopamine is associated with motivation and reward. I found that gratitude really helped me. When I was unable to do anything, I tried to focus on the small things that I was grateful for – a phone call, nature, trees, a smile – and

it made a massive difference. Doing it every day has huge health and wellbeing benefits.

High five habit
High fiving in the mirror is amazing and, according to author Mel Robbins, has been scientifically proven to immediately improve your mood and even change negative thought patterns. This is what she says in her book *The High 5 Habit* (2021): 'I see you and I love you. Come on now, Mel, you've got this... I was assuring myself that I can do it, whatever "it" was. I was cheering for myself and encouraging the woman I saw in the mirror to lift her chin and keep going.' Mel Robbins is a guest on Dr Rangan Chatterjee's podcast (see listings).

Yoga
This can help you with muscle contraction, breathing, digestion, blood flow and circulation. It's also a great way to get your lymphatic system moving. According to yogainternational.com, 'It can influence the lymphatic system, which is our first line of defence against disease. Lymph transports a range of antibodies and specialised white blood cells designed to fight disease, flow through nodes that filter bacteria, foreign matter and dead tissue. Healthy lymph is a key component of a strong immune system and yoga can help that flow.'

Unlike your cardiovascular system, where blood is pumped around your body by the heart, your lymphatic system has no pump – it relies on gravity and the muscular system. The flowing movement of yoga helps to boost lymphatic flow. I can recommend Adriene Mishler and Tim Senesi, who offer free lessons online (see listings at the end). The videos vary in length and ability so choose the one that suits you best. Take it slowly to start with and build it up gradually. If this is too much, then do some gentle flow yoga.

Chapter 7

The state of innocence

Angela talks about being in a state of innocence – the state you're in as a child before your beliefs have set in. Everything is new to you – the trees, the river, the sky. You 'inherit' beliefs when you're young to get your needs met.

The Clean 15 and Dirty Dozen

Eating organic food can help you avoid toxins but it's useful to be aware of the Clean 15 and the Dirty Dozen. The Environmental Working Group (EWG) provides a handy guide that's updated every year. This list is more of a resource to help you when you go shopping. If you're on a budget it can help to steer you towards organic produce. Fruit and vegetables are washed and peeled before they're tested for pesticides. To rank each item, the EWG gives it a score based on the percentage of samples with detectable pesticides.

Don't worry if you can't buy organic. Just wash fruit and vegetables carefully before use.

The EWG's 2023 shopper's guide to pesticides in produce:

The Clean 15	The Dirty Dozen
Avocados	Strawberries
Sweetcorn	Spinach
Pineapple	Kale
Onions	Peaches
Papaya	Pears
Peas (frozen)	Nectarines
Asparagus	Apples
Honeydew melon/watermelon	Grapes
Kiwi fruit and mangos	Bell peppers
Cabbage and carrots	Cherries
Mushrooms	Blueberries
Sweet potatoes	Green beans

Resources

Gut health
This is a big topic but the takeaway message is to know that your gut is vital to your health. It's the epicentre, the root system. What you eat has a huge impact on your gut health as well as your mind and how stressed you are. The upper gut refers to the stomach, duodenum and small intestine, which digest mainly meat and fat; and the lower gut or large bowel, which is full of bacteria and is a fermenting gut that digests vegetables and fibre. When I was initially struggling with fatigue my gut was not in a great state. I consumed fruit and vegetables in soups, casseroles, roasted vegetables and smoothies, which are gentler on the gut. I work on my gut health every day and have recently been seeing Naturopathy Cathy at Roots Health & Wellness. She's full of passion and knowledge and cares deeply about everyone she works with.

The intestines
The intestines are basically a hollow tube stretching from your stomach to your anus. They include the small intestine, large intestine and rectum. The small intestine is about 7 metres long and is the most important organ of the digestive system because it's involved in digestion and absorption. This is where most of the digestive enzymes do their work to break down food into nutrients that can be absorbed and utilised by the body. For example, sugar is broken down into glucose, which is then used to produce energy in the form of ATP. The large intestine (colon) is only about 1.5 metres long and absorbs water from the waste, creating stools that pass through to the rectum to be excreted.

The gut microbiome
As Harpreet Health says, the gut microbiome is made up of viruses, bacteria and fungi that each play a different role. We're full of natural fungi, the best-known subtype being

yeast, which is key in helping to reduce inflammation and maintaining a good immune defence. Our microbes break down fibre to produce chemicals, according to gut microbiome expert Dr Tim Spector, 'that energise and communicate with our body's immune cells, most of which are in the gut lining. These are the cells that sense when there is an infection and send certain key white blood cells to the site of the infection.' Dr Spector is a professor of genetics, author and co-founder of the ZOE Health Study. His top tips for a healthier gut are as follows:

1. Try to eat 30 different plants each week.
2. Add some colour to your plate – eat the rainbow.
3. Experiment with fermented foods.
4. Limit ultra-processed foods.

You can't extract the goodness from food without good gut function but, worse than that, you then end up feeding the unfriendly microbiome that makes you ill. There are about 100 trillion microbes in the gut, ten times as many microbes as cells. One of the main things that they do is ferment vegetable fibre to produce short-chain fatty acids (SCFA), which are the main source of food for the cells lining the colon. These SCFAs are very important in sending messages to your immune cells to keep down inflammation.

Leaky gut
There's a barrier that measures the thickness of one cell that separates the contents of your gut from your blood supply. This single-cell gut barrier is fragile, so poor diet, high stress and inflammation can result in this barrier breaking down so that gut content gets into your blood and circulates around the body, causing more inflammation, damage and disease. According to Harvard Medical School, 'Some studies show that leaky gut may be associated with

chronic fatigue and fibromyalgia.' If your gut isn't healthy you may experience bloating, burping, constipation and diarrhoea but inflammation could also extend to other parts of your body through a leaky gut. As Dr Will Bulsiewicz says in his book *Fibre Fuelled* (2020), in order to help rebuild the gut lining, eat food that's nutritious, natural and unprocessed and avoid food that may trigger any inflammatory response. Eating food that's high in fibre can also contribute to healthy bowel movements.

Prebiotics and probiotics

Harpreet talks about prebiotics and probiotics. Prebiotics, which feed the friendly bacteria in your gut, are in foods such as wholegrains, which also help the immune system and are anti-inflammatory. Probiotics contain live bacteria that are often called 'good' or 'helpful' because they help to keep your gut healthy. Probiotics are fermented foods that feed the bacteria. When trying probiotic foods maybe start with a tablespoon of kimchi, a fermented food that's already loaded with antioxidants, vitamins and minerals. It also contains other ingredients such as ginger and chilli, which will further boost your immune system and are great for gut health. Sauerkraut is also good and easy to make at home.

Constipation and toxins

According to Dr Sarah Myhill, if you have CFS it's better to avoid constipation: 'Food should spend 60 to 90 minutes in the stomach, six hours in the small intestine and 24 hours in the large intestine for efficient digestion and absorption. Longer than this increases problems of fermentation and toxins.' It's important to remove toxins from the body, and having a sauna three or four times a week for 20 to 30 minutes can help with this. If you're struggling with energy, then going to sit in a sauna is relaxing. I did this quite a lot when I couldn't do much else. As Harpreet says, your body also helps to remove toxins through your liver, skin, intestines, lymphatic system and blood. That's why getting rid of toxins and not allowing them to build up is so important. People with energy issues often have a slow or sluggish lymphatic system and skin brushing can help with this. Dry skin brushing is using a bristle brush, which sweeps across the dry skin from the toes towards the head and can help to promote lymph flow and drainage. But don't brush over eczema, psoriasis or chafing. Your skin is also your first line of defence, so make sure that anything you put on it is 'natural'. This includes deodorants.

Chapter 8

In *The Biology of Belief,* Bruce Lipton says that when the cells have a healthy environment, they thrive and when the environment is less than 'optimal', the cells falter. But when the environment is adjusted, the 'sick' cells are revitalised. So the bottom line is that it's possible to make changes and they will make a difference.

The cell and organelles
The cell is the basic structural unit of the body. It carries out many processes that define life, including reproduction, respiration, digestion, movement and excretion – although not every cell has all of these abilities. Each organelle in the cell has a role to play. In the centre of the cell is the nucleus, which is the cell's control centre. This contains the genetic information needed for cell growth and reproduction. As well as mitochondria, other key organelles include ribosomes, which create proteins that are used inside and outside the cell, and lysosomes, which are the waste bins that remove toxic substances from the cell.

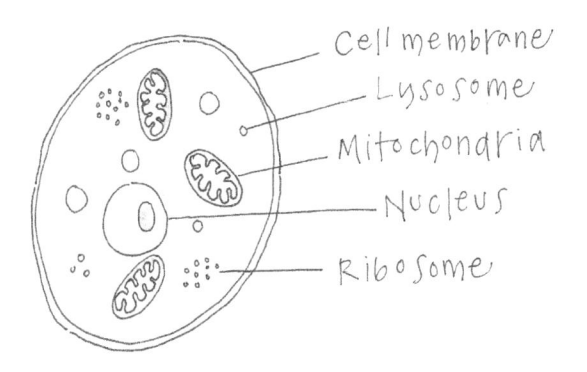

A hand-drawn cell diagram with labels: Cell membrane, Lysosome, Mitochondria, Nucleus, Ribosome.

Organelle and structures	Function
Nucleus	The cell's control centre, containing genetic information
Mitochondria	The powerhouse supplying energy in the form of ATP
Cell membrane	Encloses the cell and regulates the flow of substances in and out of the cell
Ribosomes	Small, round structures that create proteins for use in the cell or transported out of it
Lysosomes	Produce powerful enzymes that digest and excrete waste and worn-out organelles

The mitochondria

These produce energy in the form of ATP through a series of complex stages. The energy from the food we eat is stored as ATP. The whole process of storage and production of energy is complex and involves several different molecules, so it can go 'wrong' at a number of different places in the chain of reactions. There's some research that looks at where in the cycle people with CFS might have issues but it's not that clear. However, according to Dr Eleanor Roberts at ME Research UK, 'There are findings to date that suggest that there is some disruption to the mitochondria in ME/CFS.'

There are many papers looking at CFS and the mitochondria. Dr Roberts discusses the fact that the molecule CoQ10, which is necessary in one of the stages of producing ATP, is shown to be reduced in people with CFS and says that the research strongly suggests that there's mitochondrial disruption in people with CFS. Your body does produce CoQ10 naturally but there are also foods high in the molecule, including trout, herring and mackerel; soybeans, lentils and peanuts; sesame seeds and pistachios; spinach, broccoli and cauliflower; strawberries and oranges; and wholegrains.

Here are the top four things that can affect your mitochondrial health:

1. a diet high in processed food and toxins such as excess alcohol
2. nutrient deficiencies
3. lack of exercise
4. environmental toxins such as chemicals and heavy metals.

If you have poor mitochondrial function, you won't be producing enough energy to fuel other enzymatic processes such as the production of serotonin and dopamine, which are the neurotransmitters essential for mental health.

The lymphatic system
The lymphatic (or lymph) system is part of the body's immune system. It looks like veins in the body but they carry a clear, watery fluid called lymph. This fluid carries the waste products that are created when white blood cells attack and break down such things as bacteria and viruses. The lymph puts the waste products back into the bloodstream for removal by the body.

The cell membrane
This protects the inside of the cell and is involved in permitting materials in and out of the cell. It's semi-permeable and forms a lipid bilayer. It allows nutrients into the cell and removes toxic substances from the cell. It also provides structural support for the cell.

Metabolic processes
These are all the chemical reactions that take place inside the cell. One of these processes is the conversion of the energy in food to energy that can be used by the cell to carry out several processes.

The liver
A healthy liver is critical for anyone with CFS. This organ sits on the right side of the belly, weighs about 1.5 kg and is about 15 cm wide. It has about 500 functions but one of them is to break down and remove toxins such as alcohol from the body's blood supply, so it forms a huge part of the immune system. It also produces the digestive juice (bile) that's stored in the gall bladder. Bile breaks down fats and has a role in energy production by converting stored glycogen to glucose, which can then be used to produce ATP. It also stores extra glucose in the form of glycogen.

GLOSSARY OF TERMS

Acupuncture: a traditional practice in Chinese medicine where fine needles are inserted at certain sites in the body for therapeutic and preventative purposes.

Absorption: the small intestine breaks down nutrients that can then be absorbed by the body and carried to the cells.

Antioxidant: a molecule that neutralises free radicals in the body, which can cause harm if their levels become too high and lead to multiple illnesses. Some foods high in antioxidants include berries and green tea.

Artificial sweeteners and flavourings: chemicals added to food and drink to make them taste sweet.

ATP: adenosine triphosphate, an energy-carrying molecule found in the cells of all living things.

Bacteria: single-celled organisms. The body needs certain types of bacteria to function, such as those that live in the digestive tract.

Baseline: the level of activity that's possible without making signs and symptoms worse.

Blood sugar levels: also known as blood glucose levels, these show how much glucose you have in your bloodstream.

Blue light: a spectrum of light emitted from devices such as mobile phones and computers that suppresses the natural production of melatonin, the hormone that helps you go to sleep.

Burnout: a state of physical or mental exhaustion.

Calcium: the mineral that's used in the development and maintenance of bone structure and rigidity.

Caffeine: a natural stimulant commonly found in tea, coffee and cola.

Carbohydrates: a compound (macronutrient) found in many foods and drinks. They're an important source of energy in a healthy diet. There are three main types – simple sugar molecules such as glucose, fructose and sucrose; starches that are formed of long chains of sugars joined together; and then fibre.

Cell: the basic membrane-bound unit that contains the fundamental molecule of life and of which all living things are composed.

CFS: chronic fatigue syndrome – a long-term illness with a wide range of symptoms, the most common being overwhelming fatigue.

Chia seeds: a great source of fibre, minerals, antioxidants and omega-3 fatty acids.

Constipation: when bowel movements become less frequent and stools become more difficult to pass.

CoQ10: coenzyme Q10 – a substance found naturally in the body that helps to generate energy in the cells. It produces ATP and is a powerful antioxidant.

Decaffeinated tea: tea that has been processed to remove caffeine. It's not the same as naturally caffeine-free teas such as rooibos, peppermint or turmeric.

Dehydration: a condition caused by not drinking enough water or by losing more water than you take in.

Disaccharides: sugars that contain two monosaccharides joined together. For example, sucrose is made up of glucose and fructose.

Dysbiosis: often referred to as an 'imbalance' in the gut microbial community that's associated with disease.

Emotional freedom technique (EFT): focuses on tapping the 12 meridian points of the body to relieve symptoms of a negative experience or emotion.

Endorphins: chemical messengers (neurotransmitters) that are released by the brain to alleviate pain or stress and are also released during pleasurable activities such as exercise or laughing.

Energy: humans run on chemical energy in the form of ATP to carry out all the functions in the body. The fuel for this comes from food and drink – mainly carbohydrates but also fats and proteins.

Essential fatty acids (EFA): there are two main types of EFA – omega-3 and omega-6. EFA are the most important fats but the body can't make them – you must get them from food and drink, which is why they're called essential. These fatty acids produce hormones that regulate the immune system and central nervous system.

Fat: the body uses fat as a fuel source and is the major form of storage for energy in the body. Fats come in several forms, including saturated, monounsaturated and polyunsaturated (EFA).

Fatigue: a feeling of constant tiredness or lack of energy. It's not the same as simply feeling drowsy or sleepy.

Fermentation: an ancient technique used to preserve food. It's a natural process through which microorganisms such as yeast and bacteria convert carbohydrates such as starch and sugar into alcohol or acids. It also promotes the growth of beneficial bacteria such as probiotics, which have health benefits such as improving the immune function and digestive health.

Fibre: a type of carbohydrate your body can't break down, which passes through into the colon. It's vital for gut health and can help to prevent constipation.

Fight or flight response: plays a critical role in how we deal with stress and danger in our environment. It prepares the body to either fight or flee a threat by creating a physiological reaction.

Flaxseed tea: a drink made with flaxseeds that's a great way of getting your body to hold on to water.

Free radicals: highly reactive molecules that can damage cells, causing illness and ageing.

Glucose: a simple sugar and the most abundant monosaccharide, a subcategory of carbohydrates.

Gluten: a general name for the proteins found in wheat, rye and barley.

Grains: small, hard, edible dry seeds that grow on grass-like plants called cereals. Wholegrains are much better for you because they haven't been processed to remove the bran and germ, so they're healthy and nutritious and provide a good source of vitamins and minerals, fibre and carbohydrates. Examples are brown rice, quinoa, oats, buckwheat and amaranth.

Gut health: covers the whole of your digestive system – the parts of your body responsible for breaking down food into the individual nutrients needed for your body to function.

Heavy metals: heavy metal poisoning is caused by the accumulation of certain metals in the body due to exposure through food, water, industrial chemicals or other sources. The body does need small amounts of heavy metals to function normally (zinc, copper, iron, manganese) but large amounts are toxic. Heavy metals that may lead to health issues include lead, mercury, arsenic and chromium.

Herbal teas: infusions made from tisanes, which are a blend of dried flowers, fruit, spices or herbs.

Irritable bowel syndrome (IBS): a common condition that affects the digestive system. The most common symptoms are abdominal pain and cramping, bloating and swelling of your stomach and excessive wind plus a change in bowel habits, such as constipation or diarrhoea. It can be aggravated by stress, hormones and certain foods.

Immune system: defends the body from infection. An underactive or overactive immune system can cause health issues.

Inflammation: an essential part of your body's healing

process but which can lead to pain, swelling or bruising.

Kimchi: a Korean dish made from salted, fermented vegetables, often including seasonings such as garlic and chilli.

Kinesiologist: a practitioner who uses muscle testing to identify imbalances in the body's structural, chemical and emotional energy.

Leaky gut: when the gut lining allows or 'leaks' partially digested food or toxins into your bloodstream.

Legume: a plant that has its seeds in a pod, such as bean or pea.

Lymphatic system and lymph: the lymphatic system is part of the immune system and has many functions. It carries lymph, a clear fluid containing white blood cells, back into the bloodstream.

Magnesium: a macronutrient that plays a role in more than 300 enzyme reactions in the body. Its functions include helping with muscle and nerve contraction, regulating blood pressure and supporting the immune system.

Magnesium salts: can be used in a warm bath to help with sleep and reduce stress.

Meditation: a mental exercise that trains attention and awareness to help to curb negative thoughts and feelings.

Meridian points: the meridian system is a concept in traditional Chinese medicine (TCM) through which the life energy known as 'qi' flows. The meridian points are acupuncture points through which this energy flows throughout the body.

Melatonin: a hormone responsible for regulating your body's sleep cycle. Your brain produces it in response to darkness.

Microbiome: the community of microorganisms (such as fungi, bacteria and viruses) that exists in a particular environment such as the skin or gastrointestinal tract.

Mindfulness: a technique that involves noticing what's happening in the present moment, without judgement.

Miso: a soybean paste that's a staple ingredient in Japanese cuisine.

Mitochondria: membrane-bound cell organelles that generate most of the chemical energy needed to power the cell's biochemical reactions. Chemical energy produced by the mitochondria is stored in a small molecule called adenosine triphosphate (ATP).

Monosaccharides: also called simple sugars. The most basic form of carbohydrate, with glucose being the most common. Monosaccharides are the building blocks of disaccharides.

Myalgic encephalomyelitis (ME): an alternative term for CFS.

Naturopathic nutritionist: practitioners who use natural remedies to help the whole person become healthy by creating an environment in which the body can thrive.

Nervous system (NS): includes the brain, spinal cord and a complex network of nerves throughout the whole body. The NS sends messages back and forth between the brain and the body. The brain controls all the body's functions.

Neurotransmitters: chemical messengers that carry chemical signals from one nerve to the next.

Omega-3: healthy fats that support the body, which you need to obtain from your diet. One of the essential fatty acids (EFA).

Organelle: a biological structure that performs a distinctive function inside a cell.

Organic food: produce that avoids the use of man-made fertilisers, pesticides, growth regulators and livestock additives.

Pacing: a self-management technique that aims to balance energy and rest.

Parasympathetic nervous system (PNS): triggers the rest

and repair response and is part of the autonomic nervous system (ANS) that regulates the body's unconscious processes. When stimulated it can help with digestion.

Pesticides: substances that are meant to control pests, weeds and diseases but can have an impact on human health due to the toxic chemicals some of them contain.

Phosphorus: an essential mineral, the main purpose of which is to build and maintain bones and teeth.

Physiotherapist: a practitioner who helps to restore and maintain a person's mobility and physical wellbeing.

Phytochemicals: naturally occurring plant compounds that provide a natural defence system against insects and grazing animals.

Pilates: a form of exercise that focuses on balance, posture, strength and flexibility.

Prebiotics: a form of dietary fibre that feeds the friendly bacteria in the gut.

Probiotics: a mixture of live bacteria and/or yeast that help to keep you healthy. Examples include sauerkraut, kimchi, yoghurt, miso and tempeh.

Processed food: any type of food that has been altered in some way, which can mean milled, cut, packaged, canned, frozen, blanched, dehydrated, etc. Minimally processed foods include fresh blueberries or vegetables prepared for convenience; moderately processed foods have had ingredients such as sweeteners added; heavily processed foods include frozen or pre-made meals, including frozen pizza and microwaveable meals.

Proteins: play many critical roles in the body. They do most of the work in your cells and are required for the structure, function and regulation of the body's tissues and organs.

Pulses: peas, beans and lentils that have been dried. They're a great source of protein, fibre and starch.

Refined foods: foods that have been stripped and processed of their nutritional value, such as flavoured crisps, white bread and sweetened breakfast cereals.

Rest and repair response: also known as the rest and digest response. This restores the body to a state of calm and allows it to relax and repair.

Sauerkraut: finely sliced cabbage that has been fermented, offering many health benefits.

Serotonin: a chemical messenger (neurotransmitter) that helps brain and nervous system cells communicate. Its main function is to stabilise your mood as well as your feelings of happiness and wellbeing. It also plays a role in the digestive system and sleep cycle.

Stimulant: a substance that speeds up messages travelling between the brain and the body. It induces alertness, wakefulness and motor activity and decreases appetite.

Sugar crash: when your blood sugar levels suddenly drop after eating large amounts of carbohydrates such as pasta, pizza or dessert. This triggers the release of adrenaline, the fight or flight hormone. When the body has more sugar than it's used to, it produces insulin in an attempt to keep the levels consistent.

Sympathetic nervous system (SNS): triggers the fight or flight response and is part of the autonomic nervous system that regulates the body's unconscious processes.

Tempeh: a traditional Indonesian food made from fermented soybeans that have been compressed to form a block. It has a high protein content.

Tofu: a soy-based food that's made from curdling soy milk then pressing the resulting curds into a solid white block of varying softness. It's a good source of plant-based protein that can be used in many dishes.

Toxins: substances created by plants and animals that are poisonous (toxic) to humans. Most toxins that cause problems for humans come from germs such as bacteria. Other toxins that can cause problems include metals such as lead and certain chemicals in the environment.

Unrefined foods: types of unprocessed or minimally processed foods such as fruit and vegetables, nuts, seeds and oats. They're nutritionally rich and provide vital vitamins and minerals that your body needs to function effectively.

Vagus nerve: the longest cranial nerve of the ANS, tasked with regulating critical body functions such as heart rate, blood pressure, breathing and digestion.

Vitamin D: a fat-soluble vitamin that helps to regulate the amount of calcium and phosphorus in the body, essential for bone health.

Viruses: although some viruses infect, sicken or kill us, others form part of the body's microbiome and safeguard our health.

Yoga: a physical, mental and spiritual practice that originated in ancient India. Yogic practices include breathing techniques, postures, relaxation, chanting and other meditation methods.

Yuppie flu: what CFS was unhelpfully called in the 1980s.

REFERENCES AND READING

Helpful websites

CFS Health: cfshealth.com
Founded by Tony Morrison, who experienced CFS as a teenager, CFS Health provides a 'step by step holistic programme that helps brilliant people recover their health and life back'. Their vision is to be 'the biggest shining light of hope and positivity in the world to inspire people struggling with CFS and other chronic illnesses to show recovery is possible'.

The George Eliot Hospital, NHS Trust Nuneaton CFS/ME clinic: geh.nhs.uk/services/chronic-fatigue-syndrome
This NHS clinic helps to 'manage patterns and levels of activity and rest to maximise function and improve symptoms'. Once a patient has been assessed they are given a 'treatment pathway bespoke to that person'.

Goodness Lover: goodnesslover.com
A treasure trove of articles, podcasts, masterclasses and more about gut health and the microbiome.

The ME Association: meassociation.org.uk

The Nutritional Healing Foundation: nutrihealfoundation.com
From the founder Alison Holder: 'My aim is to reclaim the healing aspects of nutrition... using food to create an environment where each and every cell in your body can

heal and be happy... How we nourish ourselves is crucial and we need to understand how to support the body to release its stored up toxicity.'

The Optimum Health Clinic (OHC): theoptimumhealthclinic.com
The OHC is an award-winning integrative medicine clinic that helps people with fatigue-related conditions using a CAM (complementary and alternative medicine) based approach. It was set up in 2004 by Alex Howard, who had CFS for seven years. It works with clients in more than 50 countries and is recognised for its innovative approaches. I enrolled on the 90-day psychology programme at the clinic, which uses an intervention based on neuro-linguistic programming (NLP) and Emotional Freedom technique (EFT). This included live group Zoom workshops and one to one sessions with a workshop practitioner. I also worked with Sara Jackson, one of the nutritionists at the clinic, who was extremely helpful. I also took a meditation course with Linda Hall through the clinic.

Roots Health and Wellness: rootshealthandwellness.co.uk

The Sleep Foundation: sleepfoundation.org

Yoga, meditation and breathwork

Free online yoga sessions with Adriene: yogawithadriene.com
Linda Hall's free meditations: youtube.com/c/LindaHall-guidedmeditation
Headspace: headspace.com/meditation/sleep
Melike Hussein, breathzonelondon: breathzone.com/links
Wim Hof method: wimhofmethod.com/breathing-exercises
Yoga with Tim Senesi: timsenesiyoga.com

Helpful articles

Action for ME (2020) 'Pacing for people with ME' URL: actionforme.org.uk/uploads/pdfs/Pacing-for-people-with-me-booklet-Feb-2020.pdf

American Liver Foundation (2020) 'The healthy liver'. URL: liverfoundation.org/about-your-liver/how-liver-diseases-progress/the-healthy-liver

American Psychological Association (2020) 'Nurtured by nature'. URL: apa.org/monitor/2020/04/nurtured-nature

Appleton, J (2018) 'The gut-brain axis: Influence of microbiota on mood and mental health', *Integrated Medicine (Encinitas)* 17(4). URL: https://www.ncbi.nlm.nih.gov/pmc/articles/PMC6469458

Brain Balance (n.d.) 'Gratitude and the brain: what is happening?' URL: brainbalancecenters.com/blog/gratitude-and-the-brain-what-is-happening

Campos, M (2021). 'Leaky gut: what is it, and what does it mean for you?'. URL: health.harvard.edu/blog/leaky-gut-what-is-it-and-what-does-it-mean-for-you-2017092212451

Environmental Working Group (2022) 'EWG's 2021 shopper's guide to pesticides in produce'. URL: awakeninghealth.co.uk/wp-content/uploads/2022/01/EWG_SG-2021_Guide-Print_C01.pdf

Harvard Medical School (2020) 'Blue light has a dark side. What is blue light? The effect blue light has on sleep and more'. URL: health.harvard.edu/staying-healthy/blue-light-has-a-dark-side

Healthline (n.d.) 'Your parasympathetic nervous system explained'. URL: healthline.com/health/parasympathetic-nervous-system

Healthline (2021) 'How magnesium can help you sleep'. URL: healthline.com/nutrition/magnesium-and-sleep

Healthline (2022) 'Understanding gut health: signs of an

unhealthy gut and what to do about it'. URL: healthline.com/health/gut-health

Land, R (n.d.) 'A sequence to boost lymph flow and support your immune system'. URL: yogainternational.com/article/view/a-sequence-to-boost-lymph-flow-and-support-your-immune-system

Long Covid Physio (2023) 'Pacing'. URL: longcovid.physio/pacing

National Institute for Health Care and Excellence (2021) 'Myalgic encephalomyelitis (or encephalopathy)/chronic fatigue syndrome: diagnosis and management'. URL: nice.org.uk/guidance/ng206/chapter/Context

National Library of Medicine (2010) 'High cocoa polyphenol rich chocolate may reduce the burden of the symptoms in chronic fatigue syndrome'. URL: pubmed.ncbi.nlm.nih.gov/21092175

Optimum Health Clinic (2009) 'Chronic fatigue syndrome and the liver'. URL: theoptimumhealthclinic.com/2009/07/chronic-fatigue-syndrome-and-the-liver

Roberts, E (2021a). 'Wiped out. Energy and the mitochondria in ME/CFS'. URL: meresearch.org.uk/wiped-out

Roberts, E (2021b) 'Mitochondria and CFS'. URL: meresearch.org.uk/mitochondria-and-cfs

Soil Association (n.d.) 'Why Organic?' URL: soilassociation.org/take-action/organic-living/why-organic

Further reading

Axe, J (2021) *Ancient Remedies for Modern Life*. Orion Spring.

Batmanghelidj, F (1992) *The Body's Many Cries for Water: You are not sick; you are thirsty: don't treat thirst with medications*. Global Health Solutions.

Bulsiewicz, W (2022) *Fibre Fuelled: The plant-based gut health plan to lose weight, restore health and optimise your microbiome*. Vermilion.

Chopra, D (2001) *Perfect Health: The complete mind and body guide*. Harmony.

References & reading

Clear, J (2018) *Atomic Habits: Tiny changes, remarkable results. An easy and proven way to build good habits and break bad ones.* Penguin Random House.

Davies, K (2017) *The Intelligent Body: Reversing chronic fatigue and pain from the inside out.* W W Norton & Company.

Eger, E (2018) *The Choice: Even in hell hope can flower.* Rider.

Gioffre, D (2021) *Get off Your Sugar: Burn the fat, crush your cravings, and go from stress eating to strength eating.* Hachette Go.

Hanh, T N (1991) *Peace is Every Step: The path of mindfulness in everyday life.* Rider.

Howard, A (2003) *Why Me? My Journey from ME to Health and Happiness.* Cherry Red Books.

Li, W (2019) *Eat to Beat Disease: The body's five defence systems & the foods that could save your life.* Vermilion.

Lipton, B H (2015) *The Biology of Belief: Unleashing the power of consciousness, matter & miracles.* Hay House.

Mackesy, C (2019) *The Boy, the Mole, the Fox and the Horse.* Ebury Press

Millen, R (2021) *Burnout's a B*tch!: A 6-week recipe and lifestyle plan to reset your energy.* Mitchell Beazley.

Myhill, S (2017) *Diagnosis and Treatment of Chronic Fatigue Syndrome and Myalgic Encephalitis: It's mitochondria, not hypochondria.* Hammersmith Health Books.

Nestor, J (2020) *Breath: The new science of a lost art.* Penguin Life.

Pert, C B (1999) *Molecules of Emotion: Why you feel the way you do.* Simon & Schuster UK.

Robbins, M (2021) *The High 5 Habit: Take control of your life with one simple habit.* Hay House UK.

Robbins, T (2022) *Life Force: How new breakthroughs in precision medicine can transform the quality of your life & those you love.* Simon & Schuster UK.

Rossi, M (2019) *Eat Yourself Healthy: An easy-to-digest guide to health and happiness from the inside out.* Penguin Life

Ruscio, M (2018) *Healthy Gut, Healthy You: The personalized* plan to transform your health from the inside out. The Ruscio Institute.

Spector, T (2022) *Food for Life: The new science of eating well*. Jonathan Cape.

Whitecloud, W (2019) *Secrets of Natural Success: Five steps to unlocking your genius*. Animal Dreaming Publishing.

Worton, H (2019) *If Trees Could Talk: Life lessons from the wisdom of the woods*. Tribal Publishing.

Helpful podcasts and podcast episodes

Dr Rangan Chatterjee: Feel Better, Live More
Dr Tim Spector: ZOE Science & Nutrition
Dr Mark Hyman: The Doctor's Farmacy
Mel Robbins: The Mel Robbins Podcast
The Ultimate Health Podcast: 'How to reprogram your subconscious mind', with Dr Bruce Lipton
The Chronic Illness Recovery Podcast: Episode 23, 'How to stop pushing and crashing'. URL: cfshealth.com/podcasts/the-chronic-illness-recovery-podcast/episodes/2147839092

Helpful TED talks

Brené Brown (2012) 'The power of vulnerability'. URL: ted.com/talks/brene_brown_the_power_of_vulnerability/comments

ACKNOWLEDGEMENTS

I have so many people to thank who have helped me on my journey to write this book. My family come at the top of this list because they have been my rocks, my supporters, my carers. My husband, Anthony, who has been through all the highs and lows with me, has always believed in my abilities. Whatever course I've taken, work I've undertaken, business ideas I've had, he has been my number one supporter and fan, shouting from the rooftops. When I talked about writing this book, he thought it was a brilliant idea and would help so many people who were struggling. I want to thank him for spending hours reading through drafts and giving me constructive feedback. My dad has also been amazing at giving me guidance and help with this book and I thank him dearly. My mum, who passed away eight years ago, was an excellent cook who cooked from scratch every night and taught me to appreciate what good home cooking was all about. My two children Nick and Georgie have listened, read, given me feedback and hugs when I needed them and both continue to inspire me. Their genuine joy about the book and encouragement has helped me to keep writing.

I'd like to thank all my friends who have supported me through this process, whether that was via a phone call, a message, an offer of food or dropping in to chat to make sure I was still alive! They've helped me to have fun, laugh, chat and exercise. You know who you are and I'm truly grateful to each one of you.

I'd also like to thank the following people for taking

the time to read a draft of the book and give me helpful and insightful feedback: in addition to my dad Jim and Anthony I would also like to thank Nick Jones, Georgina Jones, Imogen Lee, Emma Firth, Debbie Howe, Cheryl White, Lynn Redwood, Sally Tomlinson, Cathy Young, Cathie Kelly, Amanda Fawcett, Kasia Lewis, Angela Jackson, Sarah Jackson, Kerry Preston-Jones, Professor Patel and Lesley Pierce. My dad Jim has also been amazing at giving me guidance and help; he has read every word several times!

I want to say a huge thank you to my dear friend and artist Lynn Redwood (Instagram: @lynnredwoodart) for her superb, unique drawings. She has spent many hours producing these fabulous drawings that so beautifully portray many aspects of the book but particularly the characters, which she has bought to life in her own style and have transformed the book into something truly wonderful. I'd also like to thank her for her suggestions and feedback.

This book would never have happened without my wonderful publishers, The Right Book Company. My editor, Beverley Glick, has remained calm and supportive all the way through with her wonderful guidance; publishing director Sue Richardson had faith in me right from the beginning; and thanks to marketing and client services director Paul East for all his input. Also, thanks to the Right Book Buddies who have been with me throughout the whole process with their helpful hints and tips and kept me accountable: Amy Rowlinson, Chantal Cornelius, Catherine McGuire, Heather Wright and Sue Richardson.

I'd like to thank a few key organisations and people who changed my trajectory to recovery, for which I am truly grateful: the Nutritional Healing Foundation and its founders Ali Holden and Lesley Pierce; the Optimum Health Clinic, particularly its founder Alex Howard and nutritionist Sara Jackson, plus the 90-day psychology programme; Linda Hall's meditations; gut health expert

Acknowledgements

Sarah Otto; Dr Will Bulsiewicz; Tony Robbins; William Whitecloud; CFS Health and its founder Toby Morrison; Adriene and Tim Senesi for their free online yoga; Georgie Gladwyn and her live online Pilates; the CFS NHS clinic at Nuneaton; and Melike for her breathing expertise.

I'd like to thank the people at Launch for helping me to create and build the website that supports this book (launch-agency.co.uk).

And thanks to the people I follow: Dr Rangan Chatterjee, Dr William Li, Dr Mark Hyman, Mel Robbins, Live Three Sixty, Charlie Mackesy, Naturopathy Cathy, Dr Daryl Gioffre, Dr Tim Spector, Dr Megan Rossi, the Nutritional Healing Foundation, CFS Health, Amanda Hamilton and Dr Gemma Newman.

ABOUT THE AUTHOR

Charlotte Jones (MCSP, NHF Dip, CertEd) is a physiotherapist, lecturer, registered nutritionist, author and graduate of the Nutritional Healing Foundation. She has also completed several psychology programmes focusing on the power of the mind.

As a result of navigating chronic fatigue syndrome twice, followed by long Covid, she has extensive knowledge about the connection between food, the body and the mind.

Her philosophy centres around giving hope to those who are struggling with long-term fatigue and empowering them with self-tested tools that will support their recovery.

www.nutrition2energise.com